BODY ENGINEERING

BODY
ENGINEERING

How to Reinvent the Way You Look and Feel

John Abdo and
Kenneth A. Dachman, Ph.D.

A PERIGEE BOOK

The exercise programs contained herein are intended for persons in good health. Before beginning these or any other exercise programs, it is essential to obtain the approval and recommendations of your physician.

A Perigee Book
Published by The Berkley Publishing Group
200 Madison Avenue
New York, NY 10016

Copyright © 1997 by John Abdo and Kenneth A. Dachman
Book design by Irving Perkins Associates.
Cover design by Peter Mills
Front-cover photographs: (background) Nick Dolding/Tony Stone Images, (foreground) David Hanover/Tony Stone Images.
Interior photographs by Vito Palmisano
Interior illustrations by Donald Abdo

First edition: May 1997

Published simultaneously in Canada.

The Putnam Berkley World Wide Web site address is
http://www.berkley.com

Library of Congress Cataloging-in-Publication Data
Abdo, John.
    Body engineering : how to reinvent the way you look and feel /
John Abdo and Kenneth A. Dachman. — 1st ed.
      p.   cm.
    "A Perigee book."
    ISBN 0-399-52294-8
    1. Exercise. 2. Physical fitness. 3. Nutrition. I. Dachman,
Ken. II. Title.
RA781.A19   1997
613.7—dc21   96-54849
                                                        CIP

Printed in the United States of America

10 9 8 7 6 5 4 3 2 1

To my father, for showing me the way. And my mother, for keeping the faith. I love you both.

—J.A.

To Bill Connell and Paul (Griz) Thompson, who taught me the meaning of friendship.

—K.D.

Contents

Acknowledgments

My heartfelt gratitude to Joe Weider, chairman of Weider Health and Fitness, who literally molded the shape of the fitness industry. Thank you, Joe, for your steadfast support and valued guidance.

Thanks also to Dr. Bob Goldman, my good friend and colleague. Bob's enormous contribution to sports medicine theory and practice as founder of the National Academy of Sports Medicine has had a profound impact on fitness trainers and researchers around the globe.

And to Saul Kent, president of the Life Extension Foundation, for showing us the way to the Fountain of Youth.

—John Abdo

I want to thank my brothers for their many contributions to my life and livelihood.

Carey, my elder sibling, believed in me and took substantial risks on my behalf when I was just beginning to cut my teeth.

Ron is at the center of some of my happiest memories. He nursed me through some of the darkest days of my life and later became my trusted friend and mentor. I have always taken pride in being his "little" brother.

And then there's Mike, my closest confidant. We spend hours on the phone in wistful contemplation of the world's (or our) gravest problems. Sometimes we just indulge in idle chatter. Whatever the subject, our conversations have become an integral part of my day, and life without them—or his companionship—is inconceivable.

—Ken Dachman

BODY ENGINEERING

Introduction

The average American, of any age, of either sex, is in deplorable physical shape. We are weaker and fatter than our ancestors. We can't work nearly as hard or for nearly as long as they did. We've got much higher cholesterol levels, much less muscle mass. Our bones are more brittle, our joints less elastic. Worst of all, our bodies are growing older much faster than they did three generations ago. Middle age, in terms of physical capacity, now starts at twenty-six. Our grandparents didn't reach that stage of deterioration until age forty.

Our ancestors had to be fit just to stay alive. Not long ago, the typical American's workday consisted of twelve to fourteen hours of hard labor. Today, millions earn their living at jobs that require no lifting, climbing, walking, digging, carrying, or any strenuous physical activity. We have no need to chase our food through mile-high canyons or build our homes with our bare hands. We can complain all we want about traffic and hectic schedules, but most of us find ourselves with a great deal of spare time. On the average we spend twenty-one hours a week watching television. Whatever we're doing away from the couch and the remote control, we're apparently not paying much attention to our bodies.

Cardiovascular failure and other disorders directly related to obesity or the lack of exercise are responsible for more than half the deaths in the United States. If these causes of death could be eliminated (and many can), our average life span would increase by seven years.

The skeletal infrastructure that holds us upright has degenerated to the point where 80 percent of us experience lower back pain.

Chronic fatigue, a malady unheard-of until recently, prevents tens of thousands of us from completing simple daily tasks. One result of this disorder can be the loss of muscle mass and, consequently, a severe decline in strength and endurance.

One of six American children is incapable of meeting even the most lenient minimum physical fitness standards.

I have a computer full of these depressing statistics, but there is hope; we're not doomed.

Most of the deterioration is reversible. We can regain our strength and vigor, cleanse our muddy bloodstreams, clear our minds, reinforce our frames, and rejuvenate our dormant or damaged tissue.

Our need for improvement is so obvious that a huge health and fitness industry has established a formidable presence in the U.S. marketplace.

Bookstore shelves buckle beneath an avalanche of health and fitness books. There are dozens of health and fitness magazines. We can view hundreds of fitness videos featuring ex-jocks, ex-drill sergeants, models, actresses, and exercise gurus of all ages, shapes, and sizes. We can listen to audiotapes. We can enrich, supplement, control, or turbocharge our diets with pills, powders, and potions. We can spray our tongues with chocolate mist and convince our brains that we've just mainlined a kilo of fudge. We can join health clubs, spend our vacations at spas and boot camps, hire personal trainers. We can buy machines—thigh masters and belly busters; skiing simulators, stationary bikes, treadmills, stair climbers. We can climb concrete mountains or row miles down simulated rivers. We can be hypnotized, aerobicized, nutrasized, pulverized, or jazzercized.

With so many resources available, an annoying paradox presents itself: Why aren't we fit? Why aren't we the fittest people on earth?

The reasons that health and fitness programs fail more often than not are easy to identify but difficult to overcome. Some programs are shortsighted; their benefits vanish as quickly as they accrue. Some are too tightly focused, concentrated on a narrow band of the fitness spectrum. Some are too dogmatic, demanding a "my way or the highway" code of conduct. Most are simply unrealistic, viable perhaps in a remote monastery or foreign legion outpost, but completely impractical in twenty-first-century America.

This is not to say that nothing works, ever. Sometimes, though certainly not often enough, a novice health seeker becomes a true believer in a fitness approach that happens to be a perfect blend of exactly what he or she needs.

Unfortunately, one-size-fits-all regimens rarely produce significant results within any meaningful cross section of our wildly diverse society. A program that matches one person's schedule and tastes is an impossible nightmare for another.

A more common failing of many diet and exercise regimens is their reliance on deprivation and discomfort. The salesman who begins each day at the Highway 12 Diner resents giving up his bear claw. The working mom who must have her kids ready for the 7 A.M. school bus is simply not going to leave her warm bed at dawn to run four miles before the "real day" begins.

The major deficiency of most current health and fitness programs is that they *are* programs and are often inflexible.

Their main features include:

Instructions we must follow
Lists of foods we must eat
A schedule we must keep
A determined attitude we must maintain
A level of pain we must endure
A routine we must adopt
Behavior we must change
Goals we must reach
Inconveniences we must ignore
Gear we must buy
People and places we must avoid

Not many of us can live very happily for very long in a regimented program. Few of us will try. As soon as we discover the pleasure we experience whenever we violate one of the program's taboos, our rebellion begins. We give up and go back to our old, bad habits. Soon we are free. That program thing? That book? That woman in the leotard with the annoying smile? History. Who wants to live to be ninety if it costs you the equivalent of three decades in fitness prison?

Unfortunately, too many of us attribute our inability to achieve our fitness goals to weaknesses within ourselves rather than to the shortcomings of a program. The ensuing loss of self-esteem frequently leads to depression, despair, and the unwillingness to try again.

Let's forget about programs.

There's a better way to reach any level of fitness you desire. It's not a program, it's a process—a continuous, integrated, systematic series of decisions and actions shaped entirely by your needs and your lifestyle. Its only rules are rules that you establish—and change as your life changes. And this process works. The evidence is all around you.

The Engineering Approach to Total Fitness

Our world is blessed with countless marvels of engineering. Cathedrals, causeways, calliopes, computer systems; space stations, spaghetti strainers, spandex; roller skates and roller coasters; the Panama Canal, the Pez dispenser—every material object, large or small, simple or complex, spectacular or silly, is the end product of the same centuries-old design and construction process.

Engineering, in one form or another, is the essential catalyst in transforming concept into reality. The visualization, planning, and implementation principles upon which the science of engineering is based are ideally suited for the creation of an effective, practical health and fitness *process*.

This "Body Engineering" process will enable you to design, execute, modify, and maintain a personal fitness plan you can live with (not live by) for as long as you live. The process provides a flexible framework within boundaries that you set. The only rules, aside from the laws of nature, are your rules; the only goals are goals that you deem worthwhile. You decide how your new body should look and feel and move, and you determine how that vision becomes substance. I will provide all the information, training, and advice you'll need, but you will control every aspect of the process.

The best engineers know that success in their profession demands a subtle blend of science and art. Creativity, innovation, and even a streak of craziness have as much to do with the value of a finished product as the materials and techniques used in its construction. I'll supply the math, physics, thermodynamics, chemistry, kinesiology, and other "hard" facts you'll need, and I'll show you how to acquire the visualization skills engineers use to see and manipulate objects that don't yet exist.

I'll also share the most relevant health and fitness information I've accumulated over the years.

Engineering is what scientists call a "contingent" process—an open-ended effort subject to any number of unforeseen complications and disruptive influences. In engineering, trial and error is the norm, not the exception.

No design becomes a finished product if the raw materials needed for its construction are unavailable or prohibitively expensive; and no engineering project is ever launched unless its benefits clearly exceed its costs. I'll provide an extensive catalog of the materials and techniques available for your self-reconstruction project, and I'll demonstrate how to calculate the costs and rewards associated with each element of your process.

Unless several essential standards have been met, an engineering effort can't be considered complete or successful. Aesthetics (how the product looks), functionality (what it does), operational efficiency (how well it does what it does), and ease of maintenance are among the measures typically used to determine how effectively an engineer has performed. Similarly, I'll suggest measures and standards you can use to evaluate the results of your Body Engineering process.

The overall state of well-being that I call *ultimate fitness* is built on a foundation of cardiovascular endurance, muscular strength, flexibility, proper body weight and composition, and several mental or emotional components: the ability to relax, concentrate, manage stress, express self-confidence, increase mental acuity, and exercise discipline. The progress charts I've included will assist you in determining where you are in the process, help you pinpoint what's working (and how well), and identify what needs to be changed.

In 1828 the British Institute of Civil Engineering defined engineering as "the art of directing the great sources of power in nature for the good of humankind." I believe that the Body Engineering process will enable you to channel your powerful inner resources to achieve a better, longer, happier, more active life. You'll find Body Engineering to be a challenging and invigorating vehicle for change, with amazing benefits that will last as long as you do.

Your drawing board awaits.

CHAPTER ONE

Structural Renovation

Your Body and How It Works

The human body is an incredible machine, blessed with amazing power sources, lightning-quick communication channels, its own pharmacy, chemical plant, and amusement park, an ultra-sophisticated data processing center, flawless propulsion mechanisms, and a huge capacity for work and play.

It doesn't matter if indifference, neglect, or flat-out abuse has weakened your body's structures or disrupted its functions. Years of damage and decay can often be reversed within weeks or months. (Elevating your body's performance from an adequate to a superior level requires even less time.) If you begin with a respectful appreciation of your body's infrastructure and capabilities, you will experience no difficulty in creating an engineering plan that recognizes and takes advantage of the basic design elements that nature has provided.

Just as an engineer concentrates on restoring a solid foundation and a sturdy infrastructure when rehabilitating a frayed but classic brownstone, you must begin your reconstruction process by focusing on your body's core structures and fundamental operations. This "start at the critical center" concept isn't at all radical—it's based on traditional engineering principles and common sense.

When you improve the efficiency and work capacity of your vital internal mechanisms, you generate a long-term chain reaction that leads, inevitably, to significant improvements in external factors such as performance and appearance. Most important, this "inside-out" approach ensures that these benefits won't diminish over time. Assuming you meet some simple maintenance responsibilities, the dramatic improvements you achieve through the Body Engineering process will be permanent.

Successful engineers are insatiably curious, intensely interested in every detail of every internal or environmental element likely to impact the project at hand.

The complexity of the human body's core systems and operations makes a truly comprehensive examination of how your body works impractical. It is possible, however, for you to emulate the professional engineer's relentless curiosity on a broader, more modest scale. I've attempted to isolate and radically simplify the internal body functions and mechanisms most relevant to your renovation plans. To demonstrate how intelligently planned physical activity can revitalize your body's operating systems, I've borrowed some industrial engineering theory to create analyses that might be viewed as "time and motion studies."

The Cardiovascular System

Perhaps the most magnificent machine ever created, the heart is the body's primary power source. An amazingly durable organ made almost entirely of muscle, your heart consists of two side-by-side pumps powerful enough to process and propel at least five pints of blood through a full body circuit each minute.

The heart's right side moves blood to the lungs, where waste gases are removed and oxygen is added. Freshly oxygenated blood is then returned to the heart's left side, which moves this vital life source out into the rest of the body. (Blood doesn't flow at a constant rate to all body areas. It is sent where it is needed for digestion, movement, sexual response, etc.)

The blood vessels of your circulatory system form the body's transportation network. Blood leaving your heart's left ventricle carries nutrients and oxygen—sources of the body's raw materials and energy. Muscular elastic vessels called *arteries* distribute blood to tissues and organs. The large arteries near the heart branch out many times, growing smaller and more numerous until they become *capillaries*—microscopic exchange media from which body tissues absorb blood's nutrients and oxygen.

On the return trip to the heart, tiny vessels called *venules* reverse the distribution process. Venules merge and gradually grow larger, collecting waste as they become veins. These veins move blood through waste management organs (such as the liver) and eventually return the blood to the heart's right side, where the cardiovascular cycle begins all over again.

Cardiovascular diseases are the cause of almost one-third of all deaths in the United States, so strengthening and reconditioning your heart and circulatory network should be given a high priority as you plan your Body Engineering process. Medical experts and health professionals long ago began prescribing exercise as an effective preventive measure in the treatment of cardiovascular disorders.

Even at rest, a weak heart must pump quickly and frequently to maintain adequate blood flow. This constant need for the heart to work much harder than it should often results in hypertension, arterial damage, and injury to the heart itself. A strong heart can perform its essential tasks at a steady, comfortable pace because each heartbeat produces sufficient force to move large volumes of blood through the body. A weak heart must beat several times to process the same workload.

A normal heart rate is about 72 beats per minute (bpm). With a well-designed, conscientiously executed activities plan, heart rate can be reduced to below 60 bpm. Do the math and you'll realize that a reconditioned cardiovascular system can "save" 12 beats per minute, 720 beats each hour, 17,280 beats each day, approximately 518,400 beats each month, and 6,307,200 beats each year. Knowing that your heart works nonstop from before you are born until the moment you die, you need not be a skilled mathematician to recognize that saving over 6 million heartbeats a year is an excellent start toward avoiding the coronary wear and tear that afflicts many older Americans.

While the heart usually bears the brunt of cardiovascular disease, most of these disorders actually originate in the arteries.

The arterial walls of American babies are smooth, strong, and elastic. Exhibiting the effects of a national diet rich in sugars, fatty meats, butter, and grease—and a sedentary lifestyle dedicated to the avoidance of exertion—the arteries of the average American adult are marbled with toxic residue. When these fatty deposits accumulate and harden into plaque, normal blood flow is severely impaired. The result can be high blood pressure (the heart must pump with a force and frequency far beyond its normal operating range), blood clots, arteriosclerosis (arteries harden and become impassable), and several other serious, often deadly disorders.

A regular schedule of physical activity produces substantial improvements in your cardiovascular system. The healthy demands that exercise imposes stimulate your heart to work at an accelerated pace, increasing oxygenation of blood—and the rate and volume of blood flow. In your circulatory network, the accelerated flow of oxygen-rich blood results in a cleansing action that prevents the accumulation of fatty tissues in arterial passages.

When you spend your days behind a desk and your nights on the couch, obstructive waste can build up in your arteries. As you exercise, your heart performs like an open faucet, pumping high volumes of swiftly moving blood through your circulatory pathways and scrubbing the inner walls of your blood vessels. Regular physical activity keeps these arteries free of harmful debris and biochemical sludge and distributes an abundance of nutrient-filled blood to all body areas.

The Respiratory System

Oxygen is the most vital element of life. We can survive without food and water for days, but without oxygen we couldn't last more than a few minutes. Conditioning the system that provides this precious life-supporting substance would seem to be an obvious goal of an effective Body Engineering process.

Your respiratory system supplies body tissue with oxygen and expels carbon dioxide, a waste product of the body's energy production process.

You already know that your heart rate increases while you are active. So does your rate of breathing. During activity, your respiratory system automatically accelerates to meet the increased demand for the oxygen your body needs to keep moving. As your breathing rate quickens, your lungs expand and contract far beyond the ranges required to support normal or resting activities.

In the lungs, two elastic sacks that capture the air you breathe, oxygen is collected and exchanged for carbon dioxide. When you inhale, cells in the lungs absorb usable oxygen. As you exhale, the lungs eliminate the toxic gases. In each lung, more than 300 million tiny holes called *alveoli* provide access to the bloodstream to facilitate the absorption of oxygen and the extraction of carbon dioxide.

Your body uses several muscles (mainly your diaphragm) to suck air into the lungs. When your respiratory system is functioning at peak efficiency, you hardly know you're breathing. Activity that improves respiratory endurance is essential to the establishment of the energy base needed for an effective exercise plan.

All physical activity requires muscle movement, and muscles love oxygen. When muscles are activated, they produce heat. Delivering oxygen to muscles is like squirting lighter fluid on an open flame. The muscle bursts with energy when oxygen hits, and the body's work capacity instantly increases. The stronger and more efficient your lungs become as you exercise, the more oxygen they can supply to your tissues and the better you will perform both mentally and physically.

The underutilized and therefore underdeveloped respiratory system common in folks who rarely leave the couch is the source of constant fatigue, lack of concentration, and frequent head-aches. A weak respiratory system also explains why unfortunate men and women can't catch their breath after climbing a flight of stairs. Exercise will cure those problems, and it won't take long to notice the improvement.

The energy generation/waste disposal functions of the heart and the lungs are closely interrelated. A frequently used measure of the combined stamina of these vital systems is "cardiorespiratory endurance." The aerobic exercises you choose for your activities plan will recondition both your heart and your lungs.

The Musculoskeletal System

No competent engineer would attempt to rehabilitate a structure lacking a solid foundation, and it is impossible to develop an aesthetically pleasing and fully functional body without first strengthening the muscles, bones, and joints that provide us with structural support and physical movement.

The 206 bones of the human body are not a lifeless framework. Our skeletons are composed of living cells embedded in a rigid casing of minerals (mostly calcium and phosphorus). Despite their assumed rigidity, bones actually possess some degree of flexibility.

In much the same way that various manufacturing and curing processes strengthen building construction materials, weight-bearing exercise places stimulating stress on bones, forcing beneficial internal movement and inducing positive change in cellular composition. Osteoporosis is a withering deterioration of bone tissues which softens and weakens the body's supportive foundation. Extensive research suggests that regular resistance exercise can ameliorate or prevent this debilitating condition.

All physical movement, from the blinking of an eye to digestion to hurling a javelin, is carried out by muscles. Every body action—including the internal functions of all organs—is driven by muscle activity.

The over six hundred muscles in the normal human body come in all shapes and sizes. Each muscle consists of bundles of closely interlocking fibers varying in length from a couple of millimeters (the muscles that move the eyeball) to about twelve inches (the buttock muscles).

Muscles nearly always work in coordinated groups. The contraction of one muscle is accompanied by the relaxation of another. Skeletal muscles are attached to two or more bones. When a skeletal muscle contracts, the bones attached to it move. These key muscles must be strong enough to firmly hold the spine, knees, ankles, hips, shoulders, and other joints in place. If the muscles they rely on for stabilization and support are weak, joint dysfunction (often accompanied by chronic pain) is the usual result. The predominant cause of lower back pain (a widespread modern ailment that costs American industry millions of dollars a year) is largely due to a lack of strength in the muscles of the abdominal girdle. Without adequate muscular support, the lumbar vertebrae are constantly slipping or pinching. Most posture defects can be traced to muscular weakness. Bones and joints not held in place by muscle slide and shift from their natural positions, forcing the body to sag and slouch and pull at its joints.

To be successful, your renovation plan must assign significant attention to your body's muscles. Activities promoting muscle development and conditioning are your only access to meaningful structural maintenance or change.

Exercise improves the strength and durability of the heart (itself a muscle) and the efficiency of the lungs. Unless your muscles are capable of the raw labor required for conditioning activities, those essential benefits can't be garnered.

Regardless of the specific exercise options that you decide to include in your engineering process, basic requirements for muscle restructuring must be addressed through resistance or weight training.

Muscle strength is the ability of muscles to exert maximum force. An adequate level of muscle strength permits you to lift, carry, push, pull, and move objects—including yourself—with relative ease. Skeletal muscles strong enough to perform their natural functions are necessary for good posture and for protecting bones and joints from misalignment and injury.

Muscle endurance allows a muscle or group of muscles to repeatedly perform without fatigue. Without sufficient muscle endurance, the efficient completion of daily physical tasks becomes a troublesome burden, and sustained exercise becomes impossible.

Beyond basic strength and endurance minimums, of course, decisions about muscle design and functionality are entirely up to you. A long-distance runner's muscles are relatively small but carry deep reservoirs of stamina. A shot-putter's muscles are large and powerfully explosive but lacking in endurance. The muscles of well-trained gymnasts and decathletes are strong, supple, and rich in stamina. The body you envision creating can—to some degree—include any or all of these features.

Exercise stimulates healthy stress on muscle cells, actually dismantling relatively inert cellular elements into unstable, extremely active components. While the body rests and recovers from exercise, the body's marvelous internal systems use these active physiochemical components to regenerate and rebuild living stable muscle tissues. Regular ignition of this cycle of tearing down and rebuilding makes muscle stronger, larger, and chemically active.

Throughout its evolution, the human body has continually and consistently adapted to the physical stress our species has encountered. The "healthy demand" that exercise produces is a practical (and controllable) vehicle that allows the body engineer to take advantage of this natural ability.

For example, if you lift a ten-pound weight ten times today, and then repeat that routine for the next several days, you'll notice that the lift soon requires no exertion at all because the muscles responsible for the lift have become stronger. Your body stimulated the change in muscle strength and endurance required to meet the challenge you presented. Extend gradually more difficult tests to all your major muscle groups, and your body's natural potential will quickly become apparent.

Flexibility is a physical attribute that enables your muscles and joints to move freely and function effectively with a wide range of mobility. Muscle tissues possess elastic energy, much like that of a balloon. Experienced parents, circus clowns, and kids know that if you stretch out a balloon before you blow it up, it's easier to fill the balloon to its maximum volume.

Muscles are governed by the same principle. Exercise stimulates the elastic energy contained within the muscle tissues, resulting in increased strength and endurance. Flexibility exercises help you get the most out of your muscle, and your workouts.

Internal Systems and Controls

The trillions of muscle cells in the human body provide the body engineer with access to several important internal systems and controls. Streamlining these systems and resetting these controls improves the body's efficiency, strengthens infrastructure, and results in overall fitness. A brief review of some of the key internal operations you can influence through well-planned exercise shows why this is the case.

Metabolism is the term that body scientists use to describe the aggregate of all the intricate physical and chemical processes constantly taking place in the body at the cellular level. These life-sustaining activities include anabolism and catabolism.

Without Exercise

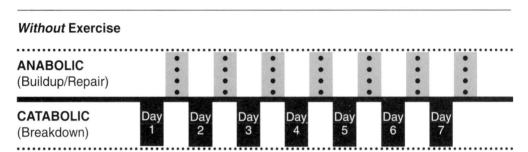

This graph illustrates the daily breakdown and buildup (catabolic/anabolic) of a person who *doesn't* exercise. As the week progresses, this person's health and level of fitness are relatively the same; consequently that person never builds any extra muscle or gets into any better shape. With the passing of each year, status of health and physical attributes declines.

With Exercise

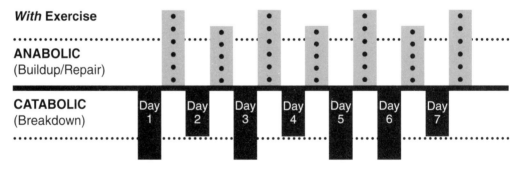

This graph illustrates the catabolic/anabolic metabolism of a person who is committed to exercising four days per week. As indicated on days 1, 3, 5, and 6 (workout days), the catabolism is greater and has increased post-workout buildup or anabolism. Even on nonexercise days anabolism continues building muscle and stimulating basal metabolic rate (BMR). As the week progresses, this person's health and level of fitness improve.

Anabolism is the series of changes through which simple food molecules are built up into *protoplasm*. The physiochemical basis of living matter, protoplasm is a gluelike substance—sticky, grayish, and translucent. Granular in structure and complex in composition, protoplasm forms the essence of your body's living cells.

Catabolism is the process by which protoplasm is broken down into its simpler, more stable components. To increase growth or strength or work capacity (or any significant change) in your body's cells, both catabolism and anabolism must take place.

All metabolic processes require fuel, and each of us has a specific rate at which our metabolism uses energy to perform its functions. When activity ceases, our metabolism continues to work—using additional calories to replenish and restore the tissues that were depleted during the work required to complete the activity. This conversion-reparation process is *always* operating, whether we are active or sedentary. An important goal of the body engineer is to harness and exploit this natural process. If we regularly expend the effort to exercise, and then allow sufficient time for the body to recuperate, this cycle of cellular change and growth causes our body's energy management system to burn calories at a high rate, both during *and* after workouts.

The energy required to perform the thousands of physical and physiological functions that are part of the body's twenty-four-hour workday is extracted from the food we consume. Our energy intake is calculated in thermal units called *calories*. When we supply our bodies with sufficient calories, various internal systems use this energy to sustain all body operations. Excess calories not burned as fuel can be stored as fat.

Physical movement involving large muscle groups requires extensive energy expenditures while the activity is in progress and fuels the catabolism/anabolism cycle that continues during recovery.

Body Composition

The often quoted formula for weight loss dictates that body weight will decrease if caloric intake is reduced and/or physical activity is increased. While the bedrock simplicity of this elementary tenet of body math can't be disputed, the formula overlooks or ignores several important physiological variables.

Most important, losing weight isn't a particularly worthwhile goal—unless the weight lost is fat. The body composition goals of a knowledgeable body engineer should center upon reducing the ratio of fat to lean tissue, not on lowering body weight.

Unfortunately, our bodies are programmed to hoard fat. Faced with a caloric intake too low to fuel its internal and external operations (a fad diet based on temporary starvation, for instance), the body will sacrifice muscle, tendons, and other lean tissue before giving up its precious fat supplies.

The body has developed an extensive network of genetically engineered survival mechanisms, and fat conservation is one of the most difficult to alter. In the earliest days of humankind's existence, famine and freezing were as common as obesity is today. Our prehistoric ancestors routinely succumbed to malnutrition and exposure to the elements. Genetic adaption at the cellular level eventually reengineered our ancestors' bodies to create the ability to store fat as an emergency energy supply.

Unfortunately, Mother Nature hasn't kept up with the times. Today, few Americans are likely to die from famine. That reality hasn't yet made an impact on a cellular structure produced by thousands of centuries of evolution. Our bodies retain genetically programmed biological "set points" which make it difficult for some of us to lose that extra ten pounds—or that extra inch of unwanted insulation.

No one enjoys being fat, and we are killing ourselves trying to become lean. Fat has a sneaky way of invading and occupying our bodies. As basic body math informs us, too much food and not enough exercise are at fault. Obviously, we need food to fuel our everyday functions. A problem arises when we consume more food than our internal systems can burn. Excess weight, in the form of fat, eventually settles in and stubbornly resists our eviction efforts.

As a body becomes fatter, it lowers its basal metabolic rate (BMR). Our BMR is a measure of the efficiency of the internal energy-burning systems that control the functions of growth, maintenance and repair of body tissues, and fat disposal. When our BMR slows, our body's ability to burn fat declines significantly, making the formula of increased activity + reduced calories = weight loss irrelevant.

The reason that this formula is incomplete and unrealistic can be traced to the set points the body calculates and enforces for itself. A set point is a level that your body strives to maintain. When we gain fat, our fat set points rise. When we attempt to shed excess fat, the body stubbornly clings to the higher set point the added fat has dictated. A vicious self-perpetuating cycle ensues.

The good news is that exercise can recalibrate your metabolic set points and help you to build a leaner, healthier physique as long as your Body Engineering activity plan includes resistance and weight training and a regular dose of aerobic activity. Weight training is an important key to weight loss because resistance exercises provide the stress needed to develop muscle tissue. Unlike fat, muscle tissue is alive and metabolically active. The more muscle you add, the more fat and sugar you will burn—even at rest.

If it helps, visualize muscles as fat disposal furnaces. Muscles contain tiny organs called *mitochondria,* and it is within these cells that fat is burned. The more muscle you develop, the more likely it becomes that fat will be burned—instead of enveloping an important body part. It is essential to exercise for muscular development if you plan to burn fat efficiently.

You must incorporate aerobic exercise into your workouts. Once you've developed conditioned muscles with resistance or weight training, you will be capable of enduring (and probably enjoying) moderately stressful periods of sustained low-stress activity (walking, jogging, and biking, for example). Aerobic exercise is fueled by sugars and fats, but mostly by fats. Combining weight training with aerobic exercise burns fat at an amazing rate. You burn calories while you are exercising, and at the same time stimulate enough reparative activity that your body continues to use fat as fuel to recuperate from your workout. The combination of resistance and aerobic activities is the core of Body Engineering's Integrated Training Approach, a sound, thoroughly tested exercise system that makes resetting the body's fat set points possible.

It is also essential to carefully examine your nutritional needs. Generally speaking, meals of 40 to 50 percent protein, 40 percent carbohydrates, and 10 to 20 percent fats will ensure that you receive all your essential nutrients. Meals must include healthful fresh foods, and you should avoid foods laden with preservatives, excessive fats, and other harmful additives.

While the weight-loss formula (reducing calories) that many people try to follow may be technically valid, it is neither complete nor realistic. Altering body composition may involve eating the same number of calories you do now—if you obtain these calories from health-promoting food sources.

A body composition formula that you may find useful is: **Increased Muscle + Balanced Calories + Increased Aerobics + Recalibrated Set Points = Reduced Fat.** As you'll learn for yourself when you apply it, this equation is both accurate and practical.

Additionally, there are nutritional supplements that encourage weight loss while preserving lean tissue. These supplements stimulate the brain and the central nervous system to produce more energy, the muscles to become stronger, the heart and the lungs to endure longer periods of work, and the metabolism to commit more internal resources for tissue repair and fat disposal. We will discuss supplements and their role in your Body Engineering plan in greater detail later in this book.

Gaining Mass and Strength

While most novice body engineers are interested in trimming down, some of you may be hoping to bulk up. If your goal is to gain strength and muscle mass, resistance and weight training must form the foundation of your Body Engineering exercise plan.

Weight training is the primary generator for functional weight gain. The stimulation of muscle functions induced by resistance work triggers the biological process of tissue rebuilding. As restructuring of the stimulated muscle is occurring, another remarkable process is also under way—*hypertrophy,* the enlargement of tissue.

In order to create the most effective anabolic state, you must apply medium to heavy resistance during weight training. This level of resistance will place the necessary workload onto muscle tissues, causing them to destabilize, forcing the body into rebuilding the tissues, and making muscles stronger and larger.

Nutrition is an important key to gaining functional body weight because an abundant food source is needed to drive the entire anabolic process. Selected foods and supplemental sources of quality proteins, carbohydrates, vitamins, minerals, certain herbs and adaptogens (which increase our resistance to stress), fats, enzymes, and fiber all play an essential role in muscle growth.

Here are some general guidelines for gaining functional body weight:

1. Resistance and weight training must be performed three to five times a week. Weight loads must create moderate to heavy resistance, with six to twelve repetitions. Workout periods should last no more than one hour. Longer sessions are futile because blood testosterone levels will become too depleted to assist in training and recuperation.

2. Consume protein frequently throughout the day. Protein is made up of amino acids, which comprise essential body tissues. It

is important to consume enough protein to maintain an internal state called *positive nitrogen balance*. Nitrogen is a nutritional chemical molecule that enables amino acids to function as structural building blocks. Whenever protein or nitrogen levels are low, you simply lose muscle. The most effective way to achieve positive nitrogen balance is to eat protein at least three times a day. Frequent protein-based meals produce a constant flow of amino acids which will raise the level of circulating blood proteins and nitrogen, making them readily available for tissue growth throughout the day.

3. Preventing tissue breakdown, or catabolism, is very important in muscle or size building. A favorite buzzword within the nutrition industry for the last three or four years has been "anticatabolic." This term refers to products that minimize the tissue breakdown process to accelerate tissue buildup.

Although many experts claim that catabolism (tissue teardown) must be induced to promote anabolism (tissue repair and growth), specific supplements are now being marketed that enable the athlete to work just as hard—or even harder—while limiting catabolism. Consequently, anabolism is enhanced. Less teardown and more buildup is what engineered training is all about. One known group of anticatabolic compounds contains the so-called branch chain amino acids: leucine, isoleucine, and valine.

---

4. Meal frequency must be increased. To gain weight, you must find a way to boost your total daily caloric intake. But be careful not to overpower your digestive system. Rather than eating bigger meals, eat reasonably sized meals more often. This eating strategy will ensure a steady flow of nutrition, increase total daily calories, facilitate better digestion, and generate more muscle growth.

5. Increase your carbohydrate intake. Carbohydrates act as spark plugs to ignite anaerobic movement. Carbohydrates are stored in the form of glycogen in the muscles and the liver. The more glycogen you make available to your body's operating systems, the more energy you will have for productive workouts and quick recovery.

The best time to consume carbs is during the most intense phases of your training sessions. Carbs consumed during workouts will raise the sugar level in the blood, making immediate fuel sources available as the body uses up its stored supply. Immediate replenishment of these carbohydrates will help increase workout intensity and duration. Carbs consumed after workouts will restock muscle and liver glycogen stores and accelerate the body's reparation process. Carb drinks make it easy and convenient to consume necessary carbohydrates in liquid form—without the need for an extended digestion process.

6. Almost 75 percent of muscle is water. Protein is *hydrophilic,* meaning it attracts and holds water. Your muscles are made of protein, so drink plenty of water and watch those muscles grow.

The Nervous System

Cellular mechanisms within the nervous system monitor and direct billions of psychophysical activities occurring simultaneously throughout the body. Control and coordination of all physical movement takes place in the brain, where an intricate communication system relays electrical impulses carrying command data to various body tissues.

A sedentary lifestyle rarely stimulates this important mind-body link. Frequent exercise, on the other hand, sharpens and quickens the brain's movement control centers, and, often, dramatically enhanced interactive capabilities develop. The process through which exercise increases muscle strength and endurance provides an illustration of how these improvements occur.

If we were able to travel deep within our body's operating systems to watch the action during a weight training exercise, we would see that as the intent to lift a weight becomes apparent to the brain, a reading of muscular strength is requested. Within the muscles, *Golgi organs* (tiny, interactive tissues responsible for generating the force necessary to complete the lift) send a message to the brain. Electrochemical signals transmitted between the brain and the muscles instantaneously estimate the threat the lift poses. If there will be unacceptable trauma, the brain forces the Golgi organs to shut the muscles down. Lifting the weight becomes impossible. The body locks up as the brain-body connection informs all moving parts that severe injury is imminent.

An excellent (although gruesome) example of muscular response to powerful electrical impulses can be seen when an electrocution occurs. If you were to grab a live electric line, it would be literally impossible to let go, even though your life depends on doing so. The overpowering force of the electric current that would control all the muscle fibers in your hand and forearm is similar in strength and effect to the impulses your central nervous system employs to communicate with your muscles.

As the electrocution example suggests, the direct link between brain and muscle is strong and instantaneous. The more we stimulate our nerve influence to our muscles, the more muscle cells we will contract. Repeated contraction of our muscles makes those muscles stronger, not only by strengthening the muscle tissues themselves but also by increasing the proficiency of our nervous system/muscular structure link. When we don't use our muscles, our nervous system has no reason to tell the brain to contract the muscle cells. Our muscles, and our nerve-muscle pathways, become dormant and, eventually, of little use to us.

Exercise prevents muscle deterioration by constantly working muscle cells. As muscle strength increases, the Golgi organs let the brain know that the muscles can handle more work. In response, the brain contracts more muscle cells and eventually resets our

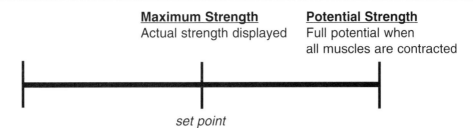

Maximum Strength
Actual strength displayed

Potential Strength
Full potential when
all muscles are contracted

set point

This graph shows the strength set point of a nonexercising person. As you can see, his maximum strength is very distant from his potential strength.

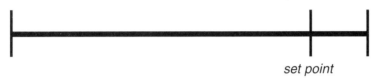

set point

This graph shows the strength set point of the same person after exercising for some time. Notice how the set point has shifted closer to his potential strength. This individual now has greater strength, power, and energy in his muscles.

strength set point. We become stronger and quicker and less prone to chronic fatigue.

Most of us have much more strength than we use. To access our full capabilities, we simply need to learn to activate and enhance our body's potential. If you exercise regularly, you can gain control of all the muscles you need. Without constant and meaningful usage, the mind-body link too often degenerates into an unreliable communication channel. Unless the control-response link is tested frequently and forcefully, there's no guarantee that either the mind or the body will be able to produce or process accurate, timely information. Unconditioned muscles, and a nervous system that hasn't seen strenuous activity since tenth-grade gym class, create a systemic dullness that, in a physical emergency, can lead to dangerous consequences.

The Endocrine System

Your body is equipped with its own pharmacy, an endocrine system capable of manufacturing a wide array of nutrients, hormones, pain relievers, and other useful chemicals. A well-designed exercise plan unlocks your body's supplies of these helpful substances.

Endorphins are painkilling drugs your body produces biochemically. Exercise stimulates the release of endorphins into the bloodstream. These marvelous natural analgesics are the source of the euphoria that superbly conditioned athletes often experience during competition.

Less powerful but perhaps more beneficial to the average person are the natural tranquilizers that the endocrine system releases during moderately strenuous activity. These substances can often reduce or neutralize the physical effects of mental or emotional stress.

Pressures induced by career, family, financial, or other external forces frequently stimulate the endocrine system to produce unhealthful levels of adrenaline or other "fight or flight" hormones. These internal defense mechanisms, which accelerate heart rate and blood flow to prepare the body for "full alert" status, were genetically programmed near the beginning of human history, when every cave in the valley could easily be concealing a saber-toothed tiger or a large angry man with a club. Today, except when extreme physical danger is indeed staring us in the face, the fight-or-flight mode is no longer appropriate. In fact, it's dangerous, often inducing angina, hypertension, artery damage, gastritis, ulcers, colitis, and other troublesome conditions. The endorphins produced during exercise influence the body to dissipate the potential dangers of unhealthful endocrine activity and to restore order to agitated internal systems.

After you've been exercising regularly, you will discover that your body recovers more quickly after each workout—even as your intensity increases. Your conditioning efforts have a cumulative effect. Because your body will be trained to produce and maintain a higher endorphin level, you'll be able to breeze through workouts that previously might have reduced you to a quivering, gasping mass of rubbery flesh. Another biochemical benefit of exercise is its positive effects on your immune system. Exercise strengthens your immune system to the point where you will become noticeably resistant to infections, flu, and the common cold.

CHAPTER TWO

Integrated Training

Combining Aerobic and Anaerobic Exercise

An Integrated Training Approach—a technique by which the body engineer combines aerobic and anaerobic exercise every time he or she works out—is the most effective method ever devised to increase muscle development, promote cardiorespiratory endurance, and accelerate fat reduction. No matter what specific activities you choose to incorporate into your workouts, combining complementary exercises is a basic cornerstone of your Body Engineering process.

Depending on the workload at hand, the body's operating systems select one of two energy sources for use as fuel. If the activity the body is asked to perform includes powerful and explosive movements interspersed with short rest intervals, the body chooses carbohydrates as its primary fuel source, triggering a process called *anaerobic metabolism*. If the activity the brain requests involves long uninterrupted movements, the body chooses oxygen and fat as its primary fuel source—*aerobic metabolism*.

Sustained activities are fueled with fats and oxygen because these energy sources are abundant in the body. Unlike steady, low-stress movement, a powerful burst of accelerated and strenuous action can only continue for seconds because the carbohydrates (stored as sugars in the body) that are being used for energy are depleted quickly.

In terms of fuel management, the human body resembles a rocket ship. When a rocket is launched, a high octane, volatile power source enables the craft to explode from its launching pad. Once the rocket is airborne, initial power boosters are disengaged and the rocket relies on a slow-burning but more stable fuel supply to carry it through the remainder of its mission. The body's initial power boosters are forms of anaerobic energy; its long-term fuel supplies are provided by aerobic energy.

When any physical activity begins, your body relies on immediate and fast-burning fuel sources—carbohydrates. If you repeat this activity after a replenishing rest, your body will once again use carbohydrates to fuel its movements. But when an activity persists without interruption—as is the case in aerobic exercise—carbohydrate supplies are depleted or bypassed as the body automatically shifts to a fuel mixture of oxygen and fat for its energy.

The sequence of this internal activity has obvious implications for the body engineer. *The body does not start burning fat until all its available carbohydrate and sugar sources are depleted.* Approximately 40 percent of most conventional workout time is spent burning sugar as fuel. Almost no fat is converted into energy until these supplies are exhausted.

The astute body engineer can take advantage of the body's fuel management protocols to design and implement an Integrated Training Approach that effectively taps both energy sources. The Integrated Training Approach is the best way to combine aerobic and anaerobic activities. The body engineer wil also use strength training and flexibility exercises as part of the Body Engineering process.

Regardless of what you choose to do at the gym, or in the den or the garage, your anaerobic activities should *precede* your aerobic workout. Anaerobic exercise will quickly deplete your carbohydrate fuel stores before you begin the aerobic phase of your training. Because there are no carbohydrates readily available, you will be burning fat continuously—from start to finish—during your aerobic activities.

Generally speaking, your aerobic workout should last at least twenty minutes, with sessions over thirty minutes being ideal. During aerobic exercise, you should aim to reach 70 to 85 percent of your maximum heart rate to achieve the best results. This is known as your *aerobic range*.

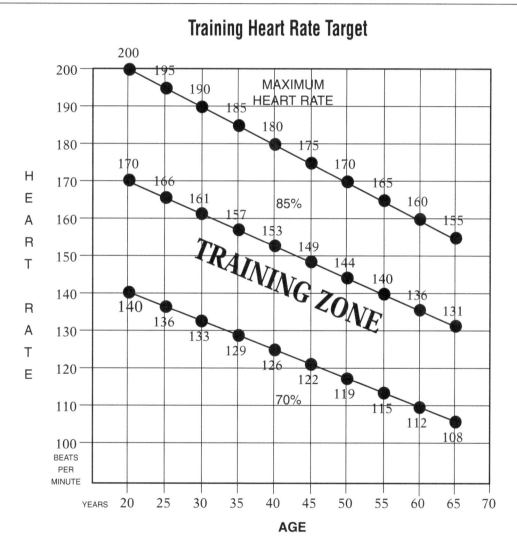

Training Heart Rate Target

Adapted from Bruce Algra Fitness Chart Series

Scientific data indicate that the amount of energy expended *after* low-intensity aerobic exercise tends to be minimal. Conventional aerobics is effective in burning body fat *only during a portion of the actual workout*. Most aerobic exercise does little to stimulate your post-workout metabolism rate. That's because aerobic activity does not stress the muscle tissues to the point where they must be repaired or rebuilt after the workout ends. Your internal systems have no need to work to convert stored energy sources (fat) to rejuvenate cellular-level muscle tissues.

The way your body burns fuel accounts for the difference in physiques between the lean, muscular sprinter and the chubby aerobic maven. A sprinter's training sessions almost always include a series of explosive body movements. While training, the sprinter will race like crazy, rest, then sprint again, then rest again. (Sprinters rest by walking or jogging.) This cycle repeats itself over and over again until the training session is complete. In comparison, an aerobic athlete may train for the same amount of time as the sprinter (or any other anaerobic athlete) but will work steadily and continuously instead of intermittently and explosively.

The difference in training methods makes a difference in the physiques of the two athletes because aerobics puts stress on the heart and lungs and rarely challenges the body's muscular system. Anaerobic exercise, on the other hand, works the muscles vigorously. During an anaerobic activity, like sprinting, the tissues in the muscles are severely stressed. The body reacts by rebuilding and strengthening the muscular system's lean-tissue compartments. This reparation period continues long after the anaerobic workout is completed. In fact, the post-workout reparation of damaged tissues stimulates metabolic activity for several days after each workout, utilizing many energy sources—notably stored fat—to fuel the remodeling.

This is why the sprinter finds it easier to stay lean than does the aerobicizer. The sprinter's metabolic rate is much higher, even at rest.

The secret to maximizing the benefits of your Body Engineering process is to use aerobic and anaerobic activities via integrated

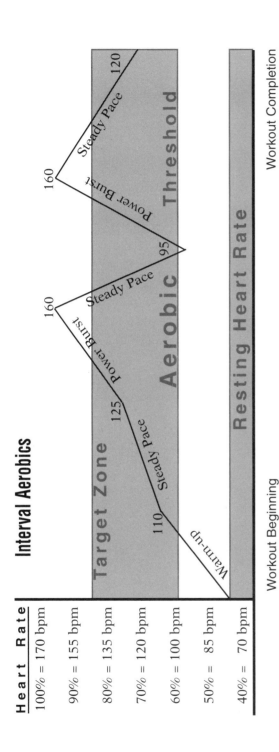

Interval Aerobics

Heart Rate

100% = 170 bpm
90% = 155 bpm
80% = 135 bpm
70% = 120 bpm
60% = 100 bpm
50% = 85 bpm
40% = 70 bpm

Target Zone

Aerobic Threshold

Warm-up
Steady Pace 110
125 Steady Pace
Power Burst
160 Steady Pace
95
Power Burst
160 Steady Pace
120

Resting Heart Rate

Workout Beginning

Workout Completion

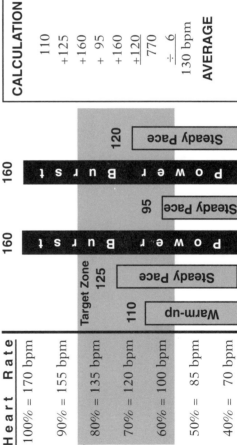

Heart Rate

100% = 170 bpm
90% = 155 bpm
80% = 135 bpm
70% = 120 bpm
60% = 100 bpm
50% = 85 bpm
40% = 70 bpm

Target Zone

Warm-up
110
Steady Pace
125
Power Burst
160
Steady Pace
95
Power Burst
160
Steady Pace
120

CALCULATION

110
+125
+160
+ 95
+160
+120
770
÷ 6
130 bpm

AVERAGE

These charts illustrate how a fifty-year-old fitness enthusiast can monitor his/her heart rate with Interval Aerobics. The conventional aerobic range (or threshold) suggested for a fifty-year-old is between 100 and 145 bpm. Interval Aerobics, *when averaged out*, enables each body engineer to register the proper heart rate (or bpm) throughout the entire workout duration, providing excellent health benefits.

bpm = beats per minute. All figures are rounded.

Illustrations designed by John Abdo. All rights reserved, 1995.

training. In addition, I recommend that your aerobic activities be conducted at interval intensities and that you incorporate some resistance training into all your workouts. You will be using aerobics to condition your heart and lungs and anaerobic activities to strengthen and stimulate your muscles. By combining the two forms of exercise, you will develop quality lean tissue that will burn fuel from all of your energy sources—carbohydrates (or sugars), oxygen, and fat.

Interval intensity means that you will design your exercise plan to allow yourself to move in and out of both your aerobic and anaerobic energy ranges during the same workout. For example, if walking were your aerobic exercise of choice, you'd employ the interval aerobics approach by first strolling at a comfortable pace. You would increase your speed and upper body movement gradually until you felt warm and loose. Then you'd accelerate to a power walk (or even a slow jog) and drop back to a pace you can endure comfortably for a few minutes before you restarted the cycle. You would continue these rest/power walk intervals until your workout was completed.

The interval aerobics approach can be applied to walking, jogging, running, stair climbing, biking, rowing, and all other forms of aerobic activity. Do whatever you enjoy doing, but—frequently during the course of your workout—do it hard! Some aerobic training devices (bikes, treadmills, cross-country skiing machines, etc.) have preset computer prompts that make interval training principles extremely easy to follow.

What you must keep in mind about conventional aerobics is that the only time you are benefiting from the activity is *during* the activity. Not much is being accomplished on the days you don't work out. In contrast, *integrated training* (combined with interval aerobics) will be reshaping your body not only when you are working out but when you are resting as well.

To complement this integrated training approach, body engineers will also use resistance training and flexibility exercises.

The Benefits

Roger Latimer, a crusty chief engineer of my acquaintance, has a unique approach to project planning. Before Roger will approve the allocation of resources he regards as precious, he requires a one-page summary of a proposed project's scope and objectives.

Basically, Roger wants answers to two simple questions: What are we going to do? and why is what we're going to do necessary?

Here are the whats and whys of the scope and objectives of Body Engineering's exercise recommendations:

What: Aerobic activity
Why: To strengthen the cardio-vascular system and improve respiratory efficiency
What: Resistance training
Why: To build muscular strength and endurance and to preserve the natural alignment of key skeletal support structures
What: Anaerobic activity
Why: To increase metabolic efficiency and to improve fat to lean body composition ratio
What: Flexibility exercise
Why: To protect joints from injury, to enhance mobility, and to increase range of motion
What: Integrated Training
Why: To increase the fuel burning efficiency of both aerobic and anaerobic activity, and to stimulate post-workout metabolic activity

Other benefits achievable through regular exercise of one kind or another include:

Increased oxygen absorption
More capillaries
A greater collateral blood supply

More blood pumped with each heartbeat
A slower pulse, at rest and during exertion
Quicker recovery from strenuous activity
Greater blood volume
Lower blood pressure
More oxygen in the blood
Reduced fat in the blood
More fuel stored in muscles
Better thyroid function
Greater glucose tolerance
More energy
An expanded choice of recreational activities
Improved appearance
Greater self-confidence
Improved posture
Reduced susceptibility to the biochemical ravages of
emotional stress
Deeper, more refreshing sleep
More and better sex

Cost Avoidance

The analyses that precede the launch of a typical renovation project include a lengthy discussion of the benefits the project is expected to deliver and an examination of future costs that will be avoided if the project plan is implemented.

An engineering team will find, for example, that a proposed redesign of an existing industrial process is an excellent investment not only because the new process will improve product quality and worker efficiency (positive gains) but also because redesign will allow the project's sponsor to avoid future costs inherent in the current system.

Until now, our Body Engineering survey has focused on the benefits associated with restructuring the body's vital systems through exercise. To complete our pre-project analysis, consider the high future costs that successful renovation will allow us to avoid—specifically, the widespread impact of the severe damages often caused by a sedentary existence.

Relying on well-established medical research, I can reasonably assert that people who don't exercise:

- Are at least twice as vulnerable as active people to dozens of deadly or crippling diseases, many of which (heart and artery disorders, for instance) are much easier to prevent than to cure.
- Have a reduced life span.
- Often become withered and twisted and immobile after the age of sixty.
- Often pay for their inactivity with their life savings due to increased medical bills.
- Are frequently incapable of enjoying their mates, offspring, or the world beyond their homes.
- Cannot eliminate the waste material in their bodies effectively. Toxins dumped into the internal systems remain where they settle, clogging interior distribution channels and slowing normal operations to a crawl. Each day becomes painful, frustrating, and sometimes humiliating.
- Have bodies that are likely to be marbled with or engulfed in fat, which attaches itself to vital organs and eventually smothers them.
- Are often sexually unattractive or repulsive to others.
- Become large and lumpy and often the target of scorn and contempt, victims of social and even financial discrimination.
- Are often depressed, lacking in self-confidence, or beset with self-loathing.

Exercise can improve the quality of your life and help you to enjoy your life for many years to come.

CHAPTER THREE

Adjusting the Fuel Mix

Devising a Sensible Nutrition Plan

Imagine for a moment that you are an aerospace engineer and that you and your colleagues have spent three years designing and constructing a revolutionary new space shuttle. It's a beautiful machine, with unparalleled power, speed, maneuverability, and structural integrity. Your spacecraft is capable of soaring effortlessly to the edge of the universe, performing amazing celestial functions in each solar system along the way.

When it's finally time to launch this intergalactic wonder, are you going to pull your magnificent creation up to the econo-diesel pump and use cut-rate fuel? Of course not. You will demand the purest premium rocket fuel available. Anything less might damage or destroy the perfect starship you've worked so hard to build.

You needn't be a rocket scientist to understand that the same principle applies to your body's fuel needs. As a body engineer, you are striving to transform your body into a sleek, high-performance machine. There's no point in building a stronger, leaner body if you are going to foul its essential operating systems with toxic debris and useless garbage. To protect your investment in yourself, a sensible nutrition plan must become a vital element of your Body Engineering process.

Nutrition is a complex science, but what you need to know for your purposes is not. Your body is a living organism. Its parts are constantly in motion and require continuous nourishment. Think of the Body Engineering process as a series of "how to" instructions for maintaining and maximizing your body's remarkable mechanisms. Exercise plays an important role in redesigning your body, but so does the food you consume.

You have probably heard the expression "you are what you eat" at least a hundred times. While it's a trite observation, it's absolutely true: The food you consume forms the substantive core of every part of your mind and body. You are quite literally made of tiny molecular particles synthesized from the food you have been eating since birth; and the food your parents and grandparents ate as well. Every part of the human body—muscles, bones, organs, skin, and blood—is constructed entirely from nutrients obtained from food.

Sadly, our society's perception of food virtually ignores food's influence in our body's biological infrastructure. Too often, the result of this pervasive indifference is nutritional catastrophe.

Too many of us regard food as a treat, a reward, a crutch, or a friend. Food is inextricably associated with pleasure and social ritual. We celebrate important occasions by going out for dinner or by attending parties featuring vast landscapes of rich food.

Abandoning common sense, we have decided that good food is food that tastes good. But taste is an erratic and usually meaningless indicator of a food's nutritional value. We know in our hearts and minds that many of the "delicious" foods we eat are unhealthful, but we don't care. We want the pleasure these foods bring. The aroma, appearance, texture, and taste of these foods excite our senses. When we swallow these seductive foods, however, internal havoc often ensues.

Unhealthful eating habits can cause a variety of problems, such as excess gas, body odor, bad breath, constipation, diarrhea, upset stomach, headaches, and insomnia. All of these unpleasant conditions are caused by eating the wrong foods, but they're only short-term problems. There are also long-term damages due to improper nutrition.

Your body needs food as a source of energy to maintain body temperature, as fuel for its thousands of mental and physical functions, and as the raw material for the construction and repair of body tissues.

Exactly how much food you need depends on a number of interrelated factors including height, age, gender, build, metabolic rate, and daily activities. On the average, women require about 2,000 calories a day to function, men about 2,500. Someone whose occupation involves manual labor needs about 3,200 calories a day; most professional athletes need 4,000 or more.

When we consume more calories than we expend, the body can store the surplus as fat. If the amount of fat in the body tissues becomes excessive, we expose ourselves to a wide range of health risks. The more body fat we accumulate, the more likely we'll suffer from diabetes, strokes, coronary artery disease, high blood pressure, and kidney and gallbladder disease.

Less dramatic than the consequences of overeating, but almost equally alarming, is the decline in general health and physical efficiency that occurs when we don't supply the body with the balance of nutrients it needs to ensure optimum (or even adequate) performance.

All food, regardless of its composition, is useless to the body until it undergoes the metabolic process known as digestion. Digestion breaks down food so that its components can be delivered throughout the body and used to sustain cellular growth, maintenance, and crucial physical operations. When foods containing products that the body can't use are eaten, the body's systems must work overtime to separate the useful from the useless. If unhealthful eating continues over a period of time, our internal mechanisms eventually allocate fewer resources to the digestive process and expend more effort trying to cope with a huge (and sometimes hopeless) cleanup campaign. When the body's metabolism is forced to simultaneously perform dual roles—digestion and waste management—internal operating systems can't perform either function efficiently.

Eating wisely and absorbing the nutrition we need to survive is both a science and a skill—a skill that must be learned and practiced. Implementing new eating habits takes time, but starting is relatively painless, and once you have established a sensible, practical eating routine, you'll find that it's not difficult to maintain.

Why We Eat

Some of the reasons why we eat are obvious, but there are other motivations that may surprise you:

- *Basic need.* Food provides the nutrition we need to sustain life.
- *Social contact.* Food is a sign of welcome, a gesture of hospitality. Every party or social function seems incomplete without something to eat and drink. Whether partygoers are hungry or not, they will probably eat something.
- *Pleasure.* Food excites our senses, so we eat to experience pleasure. When our lives are lacking in other personal satisfactions, we often seek food to fill the void.
- *Performance.* For the athlete, food is the fuel that provides abundant supplies of energy and builds strength and endurance. Food also accelerates the body's recuperation process, enabling the athlete to train harder and more often.
- *Compulsion.* Food becomes an addiction, an escape, for thousands of men and women who are anxious, depressed, bored, or lonely.
- *Reward.* Food is often used as a gesture of gratitude or approval—an edible gift or compensation that says, "Thanks" or "Good job!"

- *Fuel for your new and improved body*. A pure, clean-burning energy source is crucial to the success of the Body Engineering process.

Factors Influencing Nutrition

Eating wisely is one of the most valuable things you can do for your body. That's a simple, indisputable truth. If our bodies were separate stand-alone machines (like Buicks or snowblowers), most of us would have no trouble regulating our fuel intake. But our bodies and our minds are irrevocably connected. Our physical needs compete with numerous other powerful variables to determine how and why we eat.

A friend of mine suffered through a difficult divorce recently. He tried to eat well and exercise regularly, but his body refused to respond as it had in the past. Stress and anxiety sapped his appetite, his strength, and his energy. He felt weak and tired, and, despite this chronic fatigue, he had trouble sleeping. The trauma he was experiencing affected not only his emotional equilibrium but his physical systems as well.

We cannot ignore the role our mental state plays in nutrition. Eating when you are sad, depressed, angry, bitter, frustrated, anxious, or in the grip of any other powerful emotion can seriously disrupt your body's digestive functions. Emotional stress can and does cause physical damage. But we do know that a commitment to healthful eating will help you maintain your internal health regardless of what is going on in your life.

The study of nutrition may never become an exact science because several elusive factors impact the process. Travel, menstrual cycles, exercise (or lack thereof), sleep (or lack thereof), career demands, social circumstances, financial pressures, and even the weather can affect your body's appearance, health, and performance.

Many food manufacturers and their advertising agencies have jumped on the "healthy" nutrition bandwagon. Despite the millions of dollars spent insisting otherwise, the truth is that most of the products that crowd our supermarket shelves are not useful fuel—in fact, several contain potentially dangerous chemicals. "Healthy" has become a meaningless buzzword.

The ancient adage "Buyer beware" is a consumer warning as relevant to food as it is to used cars. The next time you visit the grocery store, direct your attention to the food labels. The more ingredients you find that you can't pronounce, the less likely it is that the product is of any use to your body.

Many of the world's largest food processors are forced to include a number of nonnutritious and harmful chemicals in their products in order to match the competition in taste and price.

The following chemicals are now routinely added to several foods typically advertised as being "nutritious."

- "Flavor enhancers"—chemicals that sharpen or sweeten the flavor of dull, lifeless foods.
- "Food coloring"—artificial dyes that are added to foods to enhance visual appeal. These dyes do nothing for taste or nutrition; they simply make food *look* like it will taste good.
- "Food deodorants"—nonnutritious chemicals that are added to foods to replace or mask natural odors with more pleasant aromas.
- "Preservatives"—substances added to foods to prevent spoilage. These are probably the most often used and most dangerous food additives. Food manufacturing and distribution often take longer than the life expectancy of certain foods, so preservatives are added. People who consume large amounts of foods that contain high levels of preservatives are excellent candidates for gastric distress, digestive problems, and other metabolic disorders.

The best way to avoid introducing suspicious chemicals into your body is to limit your intake of "manufactured" or "processed" foods. You can recognize these foods by reading the Product Information Label or list of ingredients on the food container. You will be amazed, amused, and possibly shocked by the sheer volume of peculiar ingredients that have been added to the original food.

Here's a short list of some of the chemical additives you should attempt to avoid. All are nonnutritious, and several have been reported to cause a number of metabolic disorders. My rule is: If you can't pronounce 'em, don't eat 'em.

dioxyacetophenone	undecyl aldehyde
furfuryl	propylene glycol
trimethylamine	glycerl mono-oleat
allyl isothiocyanate	turmeric oleoresin

Consumers who are not properly educated in sound nutritional principles are constantly being tricked into believing that they are buying "natural," healthful foods. Catchy jingles and attractive packages are alluring, and clever, persistent advertising often overwhelms common sense. Fortunately, as a body engineer, you'll be a step ahead of these crafty manipulators. Here are a few tricks of the trade that devious food processors often use to convince consumers that a worthless product has attributes it simply doesn't possess.

1. The bread in the brown bag trick. When bread is in its natural (and most nutritious) state, it's brown. As processing bleaches out valuable nutrients, bread becomes a pale shadow of its original form and composition. Sometimes, to convince consumers that they are buying 100 percent natural bread, manufacturers will package their product in brown translucent plastic, making the bread appear darker than it really is.

2. The orange juice joke. You aren't necessarily buying a nutritious drink when you pick up a carton offering 100 percent orange juice. It happens that orange is both a fruit and a color. All the claim may mean is that the *color* orange has been added to water or some other liquid—which, technically, does make the juice 100 percent orange.

3. The "Mother Nature even thinks it's real" line. Whenever you hear slogans claiming that a food product is good enough to fool Mother Nature, don't let these claims fool *you*. Scientists and technicians spend years in the lab creating chemical compounds that look, smell, feel, and taste like real foods. These artificial concoctions seem to be genuine, but your metabolism will know the difference.

4. The "contains natural fruit flavors" catch. You'll see this phrase everywhere, and the word that gives away the little semantic prank is "flavors." All this come-on means is that a resourceful chemist has created a substance that resembles the natural flavor of real fruit.

Nutritional choices can be simple if you take the time to read the labels on your food, and if you refuse to believe advertising double talk. The best way to achieve proper nutrition, of course, is to buy and eat fresh foods. Try to purchase food as close to its natural origins as possible. Fruits, vegetables, meats, and dairy products are available year-round in their natural forms. Other natural and essentially nutritious foods that can be bought in fresh and natural states are: nuts, seeds, grains, cereals, 100 percent fruit juices, brown rice, beans, and sprouts. The list is lengthy. Shop carefully, and you'll be eating wisely.

Adjusting the Fuel Mix for Your Body Engineering Program

Learning how food affects your body's performance is the first step in reinventing your eating habits. In addition to knowing what to eat, you must also understand that *how* you eat plays a major role in the success of your Body Engineering process.

Contrary to popular belief, weight loss is not about deprivation. (Remember that when we talk about weight loss, we mean the loss of fat, not the diminishment of muscle or other vital tissues.) You can shed excess fat by building muscle and increasing your metabolic rate. You don't have to drastically reduce your caloric intake, although you may need to change the source of some of the calories you consume. Your internal systems crave good food. In fact, each time you eat, your metabolic rate increases. Combining exercise to build muscle with smart eating to stimulate your metabolism will enable you to lose fat quickly and easily.

When you drastically reduce your normal caloric intake, your body's operating systems downshift into a defensive mode, convinced that starvation is just over the horizon. Your metabolism slows to a careful crawl, intent on conserving fat stores. Most of the weight you lose under a strict lo-cal eating regimen is primarily muscle, not fat. And you lose muscle from *all* parts of your body, including vital areas within your respiratory, circulatory, and digestive systems. This is why we almost always regain the weight we lose in diet programs based on deprivation. By losing muscle we weaken and slow down our body's operational systems. Our metabolism becomes sluggish and inefficient. As soon as we resume anything close to a normal eating pattern, we quickly regain the weight we've lost (and, often, another dozen pounds as well).

Body Engineering's basic tenets forbid restrictive lo-cal diet regimens. Deprivation is of no value in the quest to lose fat and gain muscle. The work needed to renew and reshape your body must be fueled with calories. Activity and nutrition are inseparable factors in your renovation equations.

Instead of starving yourself, eat often and eat well. Eating balanced, reasonably sized meals several times a day stimulates metabolic activity and promotes efficient digestion. When you eat large heavy meals, you place unreasonable demands on your digestive system and slow all of your body's absorption, distribution, and waste management functions. Even if you eat only healthful, nutritious food, gargantuan portions will lead to internal gridlock—and nasty fat backups at important metabolic intersections.

Eat smaller meals, and when you've finished, leave the table. Take a walk, do the dishes, read, play cards, surf the Internet, fold laundry, or telephone a friend. Do anything, just don't do dessert—until later. And when you do have dessert, go for something nutritious. This eating strategy will give your digestive system an opportunity to absorb and allocate the nutrients you've just consumed and create very little troublesome waste.

Eating smaller meals several times throughout the day will help you lose fat because the entire process of eating, digesting, and assimilation requires the expenditure of body energy and increased metabolic activity.

EATING STRATEGIES

Eating wisely requires a little common sense, a little control, and every now and then, a little treat. Your main focus as a new body engineer should be to enjoy your new eating behavior. Don't agonize over food choices and don't spend hours weighing food or counting calories. Make healthful eating a low-hassle natural part of your daily routine. The nutrition templates you'll find later in this book will assist you in establishing eating strategies compatible with your Body Engineering goals.

Right now is a good time to begin developing a practical, realistic, and healthy attitude about food. Start by respecting yourself. Set standards for the quality and value of the food you will put into your body. Become aware of the impact of junk foods on the new machine you're building. Realize that your revised eating habits are not only the right thing to do now but also an excellent investment for your future. Come to terms with the fact that if you want to feel and look terrific when you're seventy years old, you'll need to begin now to prevent or postpone the deterioration that inevitably accompanies aging.

Healthful eating requires the development of a realistic, effective meal plan incorporating nutritional foods from several food categories in proper proportion. Eating a variety of foods is important to prevent boredom and to ensure complete attention to *all* your body's needs.

Healthful eating means investing the time, effort, and money necessary for the creation and maintenance of a sound eating program. Planning meals and snacks, selecting foods, storing foods at home to keep them fresh, and preparing foods properly must become routine tasks.

I guarantee that the rewards will justify the costs. Remember, you are investing in your body—and you can expect some extraordinary payoffs in the long run. Junk food has made America fat because too many of us won't spend the time and effort required to eat sensibly. It has become far too convenient to hop in the car, cruise the nearest drive-through, and inhale a burger and fries for dinner.

Healthful eating means creating and following a consumption routine that provides your body with constant nutrition in manageable doses. Your daily intake of food should deliver the benefits you are after—energy, increased strength, heightened mental acuity, physical competence, and a sleeker appearance. Instead of eating when you're hungry, it's a better idea to eat at specific times each day—and only at those times. Try to eat every three or four hours instead of waiting until hunger forces you to the table. The timing of your meals is important. Eat breakfast, lunch, and dinner at strategically scheduled times and plan a snack midway between lunch and dinner, and again between dinner and bedtime. In other words, eat all day. But never stuff yourself at any given meal or snack time. Overeating disrupts your digestive system. If you're tempted to binge, remind yourself that you've had enough for the moment and that you'll be eating again in a couple of hours.

Healthful eating means making a conscious effort to control sugar consumption. Eating too many sugar-laden foods will cause major (and erratic) swings in energy levels and moods and drive your internal fuel management systems crazy.

Healthful eating means being realistic. There's no need to banish your favorite foods from your life. If chocolate cake or apple pie or Rocky Road ice cream makes your pulse race and your mouth water, feel free to indulge yourself once in a while. **Healthful eating doesn't mean *always* eating carefully.** Never deny yourself any food you love. Instead, manage these necessary pleasures—create room for them in your renovation process.

Finally, **healthful eating means expecting and enduring a major cleanup inside your body.** It's possible that you may not see or feel immediate benefits when you implement your new eating plan. Toxins and other waste products will be broken down and eliminated from your body. During this process, toxic particles dislodged from comfortable havens often enter the bloodstream. Once in the circulatory system (which acts as a conduit for elimination), these waste particles can move to various body channels and cause discomfort. As unappealing as this chain of events sounds, a valuable purification is under way. Be patient, it doesn't take long.

Within ten to fourteen days from the time you implement the nutrition plan you'll design as part of the Body Engineering process, significant changes in your physique and your mental state should become apparent.

NUTRIENTS

There are six kinds of nutrients that the body needs for growth, development, operations, maintenance, and repair:

1. **Proteins** form the structural framework of living cells. Your body requires protein for the repair, replacement, and growth of all tissues.

2. **Carbohydrates** contain carbon, hydrogen, and oxygen and are useful energy sources. Many carbohydrate foods also include fiber—bulky plant materials that aid digestion and waste management and reduce cholesterol.

3. **Fats (lipids)** provide energy and insulation. The body also uses small amounts of fat to repair and enlarge some tissue.

4. **Vitamins** are complex chemicals that the body requires for sustenance and operations.

5. **Minerals** are vital to maintaining physiological processes, strengthening skeletal structures, preserving the vigor of the heart and brain, and strengthening the muscle and nervous systems.

6. **Water** increases blood volume, transports nutrients, comprises approximately two-thirds of muscular tissue, eliminates waste, and regulates body temperature. You lose about four pints a day via body functions such as respiration, perspiration, and elimination. It is essential, therefore, to drink at least sixty-four ounces of water each day to maintain a proper level of hydration.

When not obtained from food, nutrients from each of these six classes must be derived from supplements.

Proteins

Complete. Complete protein foods are those products that contain all the essential amino acids required to build and repair body tissue. There are over twenty amino acids needed in human nutrition. Eight of these are regarded as the *essential amino acids* (EAAs). These protein compounds must be replenished frequently because the body cannot create its own supply. The remaining amino acids, known as *nonessential amino acids* (NEAAs), can be manufactured in the body from the presence of foods that contain the materials needed to compose a complete protein. The molecules needed to form NEAAs are carbon, hydrogen, oxygen, and nitrogen. Because fat and sugars (or carbohydrates) contain the first three molecules of these proteins, many amino acids can be manufactured within the body. The chemical nitrogen is unique to amino acids and is needed to make proteins. When nitrogen supplies are low, the body requires replenishment from complete protein sources. When complete proteins are not available in food, the body will attack its own protein sources—the tissues of our muscles and organs—to form new proteins. Complete proteins are available only from animal sources such as dairy products (milk, whey, eggs), red meat, chicken, turkey, and fish.

Incomplete. This class of proteins refers to food items lacking one or more essential amino acids. When animal products can't be eaten, a more sophisticated food mixture must be eaten to ensure that daily protein requirements are met. Incomplete proteins are present in such carbohydrate-based foods as fruits and vegetables, grains, rice, pasta, and potatoes.

Carbohydrates

Simple. Simple carbohydrates are foods containing short-chain atom bonds that are easily converted to sugar (or glucose) in the body. These carbs are commonly referred to as *monosaccharides* and *disaccharides*. *Mono-* denotes one molecule of glucose, while *di-* describes two glucose molecules side by side.

There are several kinds of simple sugars—some beneficial, some potentially harmful. Simple sugars enter the body very rapidly because small molecular size and density affords fast and easy access into internal systems. Insulin bonds with sugar molecules and shuttles the sugar to sites within the body where it can be used for energy. Most sugars are converted to usable fuel in the muscles and in the liver. When these areas become saturated, excess sugar can be stored as fat. If we continue to overdose on sugar, we will inevitably add fat throughout our bodies.

Eating too much sugar triggers several disruptions to the body's normal operations. The pancreas becomes weary from the constant rise and fall of insulin levels produced by the unmanageable sugar flow constantly flooding internal passageways. Eventually, the insulin delivery systems cannot cope with the chores of harnessing sugar molecules and shuttling sugar throughout the body. The energy available in the sugar we consume never reaches the body's work sites. Instead, it is digested and stored as fat. We experience metabolic sluggishness and subnormal energy levels because the body can't use its fuel.

The internal chaos caused by excess sugar consumption is the source of the powerful and erratic sugar cravings we've all experienced. Normally, when we eat sugar we feel satisfied until the energy sugar provides is expended. Then we need to refuel. But when sugar is stored as fat, our working systems never receive enough sugar, so regulation mechanisms within the body demand more. The more insistent these demands become, the more sugar we want, and the more we store as fat. To avoid this potentially troublesome cycle, a moderate approach to sugar consumption is essential for the success of your Body Engineering process.

The absorption of simple sugars, like those found in most fruits, can be moderated when the entire fruit is eaten with its skin and seeds, because the fiber contained in the skin and seeds controls rapid sugar release. On the other hand, fruit juices lack the fiber necessary to regulate sugar assimilation. Unfortunately, too many of us consume far too many sugar calories, and our national sweet tooth is creating maladaptive behavior in the body's basic systems.

Complex. Complex carbohydrates (also called starchy carbohydrates) are foods that contain sugar molecules (glucose) linked together in long chains (of up to three hundred molecules), called *polysaccharides*. These foods supply the body with a sustained energy source, as blood uptake is systematic and steady, preventing a rapid rise or fall of insulin or blood sugar levels. These carbs, because of their size and chemical structure, break down slowly, providing body energy for extended periods of time. People who include a proper balance of complex carbs in their diets can fuel lengthy sustained levels of energy throughout the day. They are also less likely to experience the food cravings associated with the erratic blood sugar levels often induced when simple carbs are consumed. Complex carbohydrates are found in all grains, beans, legumes, rice, potatoes, pastas, and cereals.

Fibrous. These carbs are best obtained from vegetables. They are very low in calories and fat, and high in many essential vitamins, amino acids, and minerals. Fibrous carbohydrates also contain high amounts of fiber, which helps to regulate the absorption of other nutrients and provides intestinal bulk so important to regularity and overall health.

Fat

All fats are not created equal. By now most of America is personally acquainted with the most troublesome members of the fat family. But there are useful fats, too. Fat is a vital body component, and we all need a certain percentage of fat to sustain life. Essential fats, or, more accurately, *essential fatty acids,* aid in the manufacturing of hormones which provide integrity to skin and other body tissue. Often referred to as the omega-3 fatty acids, many of these beneficial fats are found in fish oils and shellfish. Eskimos, a group who consume hundreds of pounds of fish annually, have extremely low cholesterol, triglyceride, and low-density lipoprotein (LDL, the "bad" cholesterol) levels. Eskimos also exhibit higher-than-average levels of artery-cleansing high-density lipoproteins (HDLs, the good cholesterol).

Essential fatty acids can be taken in supplement form or obtained by eating specific foods. The body has the ability to manufacture its own fat by robbing carbon, hydrogen, and oxygen from other molecules like glucose. However, we do not have the genetic code necessary to manufacture the bonding structure needed for most essential fatty acids, especially *linoleic acid* (LA). LA is essential to the operation of many body functions. You will want to supplement this vital nutrient if you're not getting enough LA from your meals.

Some other "good fats" you should know about are the following.

- *Cod-liver oil.* Containing vitamins A and D, cod-liver oil assists in preventing the formation of blood clots which endanger the circulatory system and cause heart attacks and strokes. Other fish oils that provide similar benefits can be found in tuna, salmon, shark, halibut, sole, flounder, mussels, crab, scallops, and lobster.
- Oils extracted from flaxseed, pumpkin seed, soybeans, walnuts, canola, almonds, sunflowers, corn, sesame, rice, and olives.
- *Lecithin.* A unique substance that contains a variety of health-promoting constituents including vitamins, minerals, and fatlike compounds, lecithin is found in virtually all body cells, and it plays a vital role in health and longevity. Lecithin also helps to break down fats, making fat molecules easier to burn for energy. Experts claim that the body has the ability to manufacture its own lecithin, but many health professionals and fitness enthusiasts use lecithin supplements.
- *Evening primrose oil (EPO).* Derived from a wild herb, EPO is a valuable source of an essential fat that helps to protect the body against blood clots, arthritis, and a variety of physical traumas. EPO is also known as gamma-linoleic acid, or GLA.

Vitamins

Vitamins are necessary for the proper growth, maintenance, and repair of the body. They play an essential role in all metabolic functions and help convert the food we eat into energy, which fuels body operations. Many foods contain vitamins, but supplements provide direct access to these vital nutrients. Unless a severe deficiency is diagnosed or your nutritionist suggests otherwise, vitamins are best taken in combinations rather than in single forms. Using single-form vitamins often creates imbalances, which trigger severe biochemical reactions within the body.

Minerals

Minerals (also referred to as electrolytes) play a vital role in human health, enhancing the operations of several bodily functions. According to experts, we need a constant supply of over sixty minerals to live long, productive lives. Minerals are largely derived from soil and rocks, and are found in water, meat, vegetables, grains, and fruits. These sources all contain varying degrees of minerals absorbed from the earth. Mineral needs vary by individual. I feel it is best to consume minerals in a complex or compounded product, unless a specific and severe deficiency is diagnosed by a health professional.

SUPPLEMENTS

According to Joel D. Wallach, a 1991 Nobel Prize nominee in medicine, each of us has the DNA potential to live from 120 to 140 years.

Why, then, is the average life span in America only 75.5 years? The answer to that question is brief: nutritional deficiency.

Americans who die from "natural causes" are actually victims of nutritional sabotage. There is a growing body of evidence that almost all known terminal diseases can be directly linked to a nutrient deficiency. As Wallach suggested in *Dead Doctors Don't Lie,* calcium deficiency alone can cause 147 different diseases, including osteoporosis, the number ten killer of U.S. adults.

Eating wisely is an important factor in preventing nutritional deficiencies, but food by itself cannot provide 100 percent of the nutrition our bodies need to perform standard everyday functions—let alone sustain the lifestyle of an active body engineer. No matter how carefully you plan, eating three meals and a couple of snacks a day will rarely replace the resources your body must expend to meet the physical, social, occupational, and emotional demands of normal daily living. In recognition of this cold hard fact, your Body Engineering process should use nutritional supplementation as longevity insurance.

Before we discuss supplements, remember that fresh healthful food is the basis of all nutrition. Reengineer your eating habits before you start swallowing handfuls of pills. Actual food must remain your primary fuel source, but it's foolish to hope that you can meet all your body's needs without supplements. Many of our modern food sources have been stripped of nutrients. We are buying and consuming foods that are far inferior to those harvested from the mineral-rich fields and forests of yesteryear. The actual nutritional benefit available from many of our foods—especially fruits, vegetables, and grains—is considerably lower than it was when our parents and grandparents were growing up.

If you were determined to gather all the nutrients your body requires from food, you'd have to eat all day, every day. That's obviously an impractical and dangerous approach, so after implementing eating strategies appropriate for your Body Engineering goals, supplement. Supplements will provide the additional nutrition you need without overburdening your body's internal systems with excess calories and bulk volume.

Because individual nutritional needs vary so widely, it is almost impossible to specify what supplements you need and when you need them. For an accurate assessment of your supplementation needs, visit a health professional qualified to provide you with a complete nutritional profile. Blood and urine tests will pinpoint toxins and biophysical deficiencies hampering the efficient operation of your internal mechanisms.

Because nutrients work together within the body, several compatible supplements may be needed for optimum health. For example, if you are feeling listless and sluggish and you read a description of vitamin B_{12} proclaiming that this supplement provides energy, you decide to load up on B_{12}. But, rather than correcting your energy-level deficiency, the indiscriminate use of B_{12} may in fact cause serious internal imbalances and disrupt your entire system. Eating well and designing a sensible strategy of supplementation will guarantee that you'll be providing your body with the energy sources it requires for development and maintenance.

Supplements to Evaluate

Supplements come in many forms—tablets, capsules, powders, liquids, sprays, gum, drops, wafers, and bars. Choose the shapes and sizes most convenient to your lifestyle.

When using supplements, always consult the label for the proper dosage and consumption schedule. Due to legal constraints, some labels cannot prescribe the dosages needed for highly active people, or for those simply needing higher than average nutritional assistance. Standards for recommended daily (or dietary) allowances (RDAs) have been established and must be enforced. Many experts believe that some RDA levels are inadequate, especially for active people. If you have concerns about supplement dosages, consult your health professional.

Although I endorse the use of supplements, I do not insist that they be taken every day, year-round. Occasional "off" days are sometimes beneficial, and if you've been consuming supplements regularly for several months, an entire week's abstinence will do no harm.

The list that follows presents some of the most useful supplements currently available. Note that some of these supplements are compounded formulas (made up of two or more substances).

Antioxidants: 2–3 times daily with meals. These nutrients are free-radical scavengers. Free radicals are toxic substances that invade the body and damage cells. If antioxidants are not present to apprehend and eliminate free radicals, scientists believe that we will age faster—due to the acceleration of normal cellular deterioration. Antioxidants also improve protein synthesis and tissue regeneration following exercise. Most antioxidant products on the market are fortified with vitamins A, C, and E, beta-carotene, selenium, zinc, ginkgo biloba, OPCs and other highly effective free-radical combatants.

B complex: 25–100 mg daily. Without B vitamins, food cannot be converted into energy. B vitamins are essential to the maintenance of an efficient nervous system, and they also help to sustain the integrity of the muscles of the intestinal tract and to enhance the health of the skin, nails, eyes, mouth, and liver.

Carbohydrates: Most carbohydrate supplements are consumed to increase energy production for the active person or athlete. These supplements can also be used to replenish electrolytes (body minerals) depleted by excessive heat, perspiration, and strenuous activity. Minerals and other nutrients are often added to carb supplements to take advantage of the sweet and sugary flavor present in many carbohydrate compounds. Carb supplements come in powders you can mix yourself, sports drinks, and sports snack bars.

Colloidal minerals: 2–3 oz. daily. All body tissues contain gel-like minerals. These nutrients are essential for vitality and are responsible for the formation and maintenance of our bones, muscles, nerves, and organs, including the brain and the heart.

CoQ10: 30 mg daily. This product is an antiaging nutrient. It is useful in the production of energy and in improving immune system functions.

Creatine monohydrate: 1 gram daily. This product took the sports nutrition market by storm in the early nineties. CM is a form of muscle energy that is stored in the tissues and released during exercise. The more creatine that muscles can receive and store, the more energy they can release. The ultimate result is greater strength, energy, and stamina.

Enzymes: as recommended, 3 times daily with meals. All the body's chemical reactions are directed by enzymes. Enzymes dissolve food so that it can be absorbed through the intestinal wall. After food particles have entered internal systems, other enzymes assist in converting nutrients into functional building materials. Most foods are low in enzymatic activity, so supplemental sources can assist metabolic activity significantly. There are many types of enzymes, each having a distinct role in digesting a specific class of food (fats, proteins, carbohydrates, etc.). Select a product that contains enzymes compatible with your eating strategies.

Lactobacillus acidophilus: 1,000–2,000 mg before meals. The health and integrity of the intestinal tract is essential for a long, high-quality life. Without a fully functional intestinal tract we are unable to assimilate the foods we eat and the healthful nutrients these foods contain. LA helps to maintain the integrity of the intestines by providing bacteria that keep toxins in our intestines under control. If you're experiencing digestive disorders and/or bowel irregularities, LA is a supplement highly recommended by health professionals around the world.

L-carnitine (lipotropic agent): 600 mg daily. This is an amino acid that helps the body to burn fat—by forcing fat into tissues that can use fat as a fuel source. Without L-C in our bodies, we may experience difficulty burning fat despite our best exercise and dietary efforts. L-C also has a beneficial effect on the heart and may increase overall body energy levels.

Melatonin: 3 mg at bedtime, 3–4 times a week. Insomnia is sometimes caused by a decline in the production of the hormone melatonin in the brain. Using a melatonin supplement before bedtime has given back sleep to thousands who have tossed and turned for years. Melatonin is also known to stimulate and reset the production of other hormones in the body, specifically growth hormones and insulin-like growth factor-1 (IGF-1). These hormones are essential for maintaining a youthful biochemistry. They maintain lean muscle, increase the metabolism of fat, and provide energy.

Minerals: Depending on your blood assay, here are some minerals you may decide to supplement:

aluminum	germanium	potassium
bismuth	hydrogen	selenium
boron	iodine	silicon
calcium	iron	silver
carbon	magnesium	sodium
chloride	manganese	sulfur
chromium	molybdenum	tin
copper	nickel	vanadium
fluoride	phosphorus	zinc

Protein: Protein supplements have become very popular, and for good reason. Proteins, and the amino acids they supply, provide our bodies with building blocks for vital tissues—the muscles, heart, veins, organs, skin, and nails. Protein also helps to create the enzymes the body uses for digestion, energy generation, and growth. And protein assists in the formation of antibodies the immune system employs to combat infections.

There are many protein supplements on the market today. I prefer those that provide all the essential and non-essential amino acids. These products will supplement your eating plan by providing the extra protein you need to build strong healthy tissues. Protein supplements are available in powders, capsules, tablets, and chewable wafers.

These are the essential amino acids (EAAs):

isoleucine	lysine	arginine*
phenylalanine	tryptophan	histidine
leucine	methionine	cysteine
threorine	valine	

*for children only

Vitamin C (esterized): 250–3,000 mg daily. This miracle vitamin acts as a powerful antioxidant. It is also essential for the development and maintenance of connective tissue in skin, ligaments, and bones. Vitamin C aids in the formation of red blood cells and is a component of the scar tissue the body generates to accelerate the healing of wounds.

Vitamin E: 400 IUs daily. This vitamin is also an antioxidant. Vitamin E nourishes cells and strengthens muscles and the heart. It plays a crucial role in healing wounds and in improving nervous system functions.

Herbs: Herbal supplements can provide a variety of health benefits. Herbs are plants packed with nutritional and medicinal qualities. Human physiology responds positively to the natural chemical composition of these valuable substances. There are an infinite number of herbs and plant products that can enhance appearance, performance, and general well-being. Following are brief descriptions of some of the most popular.

Alfalfa is loaded with nutrition. It contains protein, carbohydrates, and several minerals. This herb is often used as a health builder and restorative tonic. Alfalfa can ease most digestive disorders and help to regenerate strength and energy.

Buckthorn acts as a mild laxative, relieving discomfort in the stomach and colon. This herb is often prescribed for chronic constipation.

Burdock is packed with minerals and is especially helpful in building and purifying the blood. This herb may also promote normal kidney functions, as it assists in the elimination of harmful wastes that are normally filtered through the kidneys.

Camomile in tea or capsule form has become a popular natural tranquilizer. For those afflicted with insomnia, this herb is a safe sleeping potion. Camomile is also used as a cold and flu remedy.

Damiana—which contains naturally created hormonelike substances—is often used as a mild aphrodisiac, an antidepressant, and an aid to the digestive system. Damiana influences the body and mind with restorative properties that stimulate vitality, endurance, and virility. This herb also acts as a tonic for the central nervous system and is often used to treat depression and anxiety. Damiana is a safe and natural diuretic. The hormone testosterone provides several benefits for both men and women, and damiana is known to raise testosterone levels in both sexes. Damiana may increase blood flow to the pelvic area soon after ingestion, and it may also increase sperm count in men. This herb is believed to cure impotence caused by performance anxiety.

Dandelion assists the liver and several other organs in the elimination of toxins from the body. It is of special benefit to the stomach and intestinal tract and is known to be an excellent diuretic. Dandelion also lowers blood pressure by aiding the operations of the heart and the circulatory system.

Dioscorea villosa (wild yam) is a natural compound that acts as a natural source of DHEA, the most prevalent steroid hormone produced in the body. When DHEA levels begin to decline (usually after age thirty), the body's production of all other hormones also tends to slow down. By maintaining a healthy level of DHEA you will experience healthier endocrine functioning, improve general health, and promote a fulfilling sex life.

Dong quai is a general female gynecological tonic that is useful in treating menstrual and menopausal symptoms, such as hot flashes and vaginal dryness. It also helps to purify blood.

Echinacea is very popular for its medicinal qualities. This herb is effective in the treatment of many inflammatory conditions, arthritis, and various viral diseases.

Ephedra is an herb with powerful stimulant properties, and it has become widely recommended as a weight-loss aid. This herb stimulates the sympathetic nervous system, increases core body temperature, and acts as a diuretic. **Caution: Ephedra is very powerful and can cause unpleasant and dangerous side effects if overused or abused.**

Ginkgo bilboa has been proved to be extremely effective in increasing the circulation of blood flow throughout the body, especially to the brain. This herb is known to improve memory and all cognitive functions. It is being used today as an antiaging tonic for the elderly. Ginkgo also acts as a powerful antioxidant, preserving the tissues of the body and brain by acting as a free-radical scavenger. It may also improve vision.

Ginseng is widely regarded as the most popular herb, and for good reason. It provides some benefit to almost all body functions, including the heart. Ginseng boosts performance in athletes while balancing the body's systems to fight fatigue and stress. This herb has been proved to promote growth of the testes, increase sperm count and testosterone levels, and enhance sexual activity.

Goldenseal is known to reduce cold and flu symptoms and is also useful as an anti-inflammatory agent.

Kelp is a remarkable plant from the sea with an amazing growth rate. Often reaching heights of over two hundred feet, kelp is rich in minerals—especially iodine, which is important for the maintenance of a healthy thyroid. Kelp is used in many weight management and fat-loss programs to help stimulate metabolism. It also improves important functions of the kidneys, heart, and muscles.

Kola nut is a natural stimulant of the nervous system and is useful in fighting fatigue. It is also an effective remedy for some depressive conditions and as a performance booster for athletes. This herb contains caffeine.

Licorice has a healthful effect on the entire body. It assists the adrenal glands in producing hormones that help diminish the harmful effects of stress and fatigue. Licorice is also useful as a mild laxative and as a cleansing agent for blood.

Milk thistle is one of the most popular and effective liver tonics available in nature.

Pantocrine is used in Eastern medicine as a staple ingredient in many herbal formulations and compounds. This product acts as a powerful hormonal system stimulator, an effective sexual tonic, and a vigilant protector of nervous and muscular systems. Some advocates endow pantocrine with antiaging properties.

Saw palmetto is a very important herb for the aging male. As a man grows older, his risk of benign prostatic hypertrophy (BPH), enlargement of the prostate gland, increases. Saw palmetto maintains a healthy level of testosterone and actively prevents its conversion into a radical hormone called dihydrotestosterone (DHT), which often damages the prostate. This herb will make the aging male healthier, more active, and more sexually alert.

Valerian is a popular herb that is used to treat sleep disorders and to calm testy nerves. It can also be helpful to women experiencing menstrual cramps.

Willow acts as a natural analgesic and is useful in treating fevers, headaches, arthritic conditions, and pain.

Yohimbe assists in weight management but is better known as a male aphrodisiac. This herb enhances stimulation of the sympathetic nervous system, triggering more frequent penile erections and an increase in the intensity of sexual experiences. Yohimbine, the purest version of yohimbe, is the only drug approved by the Food and Drug Administration for treatment of erectile dysfunction.

SPORTS PERFORMANCE

This section is for body engineers interested in creating a fuel mixture that will promote peak performance. Sports performance nutrition is designed to push the body to its full potential. I will discuss general nutritional needs for enhancing athletic performance now, and the templates in chapter 5 will offer more detailed guidelines tailored to specific competitive activities.

Sports nutrition is ergogenically oriented. The term *ergogenic* is used to describe any measure that will boost performance or, in the case of a bodybuilder, appearance. Ergogenic sports nutrition is a controversial issue among many health enthusiasts because some experts believe that pushing the body beyond its normal limitations can cause health problems. I agree that some ergogenic regimens are excessive, but I also contend that, if designed and implemented correctly, ergogenic sports performance nutrition can be an invaluable aid for competitive athletes.

Let's clarify here that the label "ergogenic" applies not only to energy-enhancing food and natural supplements but to certain drugs as well. When drugs enter the picture, the athlete inevitably experiences side effects—some of which may be dangerous. Rather than encouraging you to take unnecessary risks with ergogenic drugs, I will confine my discussion to safe, natural, and effective sports performance nutrition.

We must also point out that sports performance nutrition can be a double-edged sword. While an athlete committed to ergogenic nutrition will experience higher levels of energy, strength, speed, and stamina, the athlete must not allow these expanded capabilities to induce overtraining.

A competitive athlete's demanding training sessions impose a great deal of stress on the body—a level of exertion that requires longer recovery periods. Without adequate rest the body is unable to regenerate and reassemble vital tissue. At some point in a hyperintensive training regimen, the athlete will simply stop progressing. The Body Engineering process enables you to avoid this "brick wall" effect. By incorporating my training and nutritional guidelines into your renovation process, you should expect to experience steady, consistent progress.

Sports performance nutrition is an extremely individualized, extremely dynamic process. As you progress along the training continuum, several adjustments to your eating strategies may become necessary to reach your performance goals. Each body burns fuel differently. And various sports require different fuel sources. Aerobic athletes, for instance, generally need more fuel from carbohydrates and fats than do anaerobic athletes. If you are an athlete who incorporates integrated training methods, you will require several different foods to fuel your training. Keep in mind that sports performance nutrition is a constantly evolving self-directed practice. I will show you how to design your eating patterns to complement the energy you exert, the goals you set, and the recovery period your body needs between training sessions.

Body Engineering's nutritional guidelines for enhancing sports performance are designed to:

1. Identify foods that provide energy, strength, and endurance
2. Assist in more intense and longer training sessions
3. Speed recuperation from training
4. Enable the body to assimilate all the benefits that intense training will provide

The nutritional programs of athletes must provide the fuel needed to perform specific training cycles at the highest level possible. Most topflight athletes plan training cycles that revolve around their sport's season or a premier event. These training cycles usually consist of three phases: preparation, competition, and recovery.

The *preparation phase* establishes the baseline needs the athlete must meet to ensure an adequate level of conditioning. Reaching this baseline level provides a solid foundation for the development of the skills needed to excel at specific sports.

The *competition phase* focuses on development of the specific physical traits and skills the athlete needs for peak performance in his or her competition.

During the *recovery phase* of the training cycle, the athlete replenishes internal resources expended in training activities. The recovery phase is also used to analyze progress and, if necessary, to redesign elements of the training cycle.

When athletes alter their training programs, they also adjust their diets to accommodate the demands of revamped training sessions. Knowledgeable athletes constantly revise their eating strategies to find the combination of food and supplements that provides optimum strength and energy.

A body engineer determined to achieve maximum benefits from the sports performance training process should take a similar approach. The effectiveness of your eating patterns should be reflected in your body's performance. If it's not, something needs to be changed.

Eating for sports performance often requires more calories than you might expect. Hunger cannot be used as a good indicator of your body's nutritional needs because your body's sensitivity to hunger will sometimes shut down when you are training hard. If designed and scheduled correctly, exercise should stimulate a reasonable appetite. You'll automatically start to crave good foods with solid nutrition, and you'll enjoy eating appropriate quantities. Don't be afraid to eat when you're training intensely, but, of course, don't overdo it.

Sports performance nutrition is an essential tool for the construction of an athletic body. Pay close attention to your food intake and take the time to eat wisely while you are training. You'll be pleased with the results.

A successful body renovation effort must include the design and implementation of an effective and realistic eating strategy. Consistent reliance on defective or deficient fuel sources can dilute or negate the benefits of exercise and jeopardize the entire Body Engineering process.

Your body's essential functions require clean, high-grade energy. Except for safety-driven limits on fats and sugars, there are really no restrictions on the specific foods and supplements you can blend to meet these needs.

As I've stressed repeatedly, engineering is a creative "whatever works" discipline. You can eat well with minimal effort and a pinch of imagination. Experiment freely within the broad nutritional guidelines you'll find in chapter 5. Explore the hundreds of health-oriented cookbooks and menu planners available at your local public library or bookstore. Spend as much time as it takes to develop a well-balanced and personally satisfying eating strategy.

Food supplies both energy and raw materials for the Body Engineering process. How well you manage this elemental resource (don't worry, I'll show you how) will dictate how quickly you'll reach your renovation goals.

CHAPTER FOUR

Surveying the Baseline

Determining the Shape You Are In

An industrial engineering team commissioned to redesign a factory's production lines typically spends its first several weeks on the job evaluating every aspect of the plant's existing systems and operations. Before the team can begin restructuring the current manufacturing process, its members want—and need—the answers to hundreds of questions. What works well? What doesn't? How much of the plant's current infrastructure is viable? What equipment can be modified or salvaged? What are the building's physical limitations?

Relentless inquiry and intense observation continue until every significant detail needed to plan the project has been uncovered and illuminated.

This baseline data, when correctly analyzed, provides an accurate assessment of the project's scope (what must be done) and benchmark levels to measure the completed project's value (objective confirmation of improvement).

The self-assessment tests you'll find in this chapter form Body Engineering's baseline surveys. Evaluation of your body's present condition and capabilities will supply you with a clear picture of where you are now in relation to your desired fitness level, and offer a glimpse of what your body can become.

As you move through the assessment phase, it's important to keep in mind that the tests you'll be taking aren't being graded. These tests are investigative exercises, akin to an eye exam, not an algebra final. There are no pass/fail criteria. As you may have noticed, your body is distinctly different from the body of your neighbor, your boss, or your favorite sports star. So are your fitness goals, your lifestyle, and your vision of the future.

The information you glean from your self-assessments is for your use only. What you learn will become the starting point for a highly personalized renovation plan—a process blueprint that meets your individual needs. The purpose of the Body Engineering process is to provide specific solutions to specific problems. Obviously, clear identification of problem areas is crucial to the success of your efforts. As you complete the assessments, record your results on the table below. Your scores will be useful later in selecting the right fitness and nutrition plan for your particular needs.

Some experts base definitions of fitness on rigid mathematical formulas measuring heart rate, work capacity, fat-to-weight ratios, and other similar calculations. I don't. While recognizing the value of objective standards (and invoking them when necessary), Body Engineering's concept of fitness is broader, more practical, and certainly more realistic than numerical standards. I believe that being fit means being comfortable with your strength and energy levels, the way you move, the way you look, and the way you feel about yourself. In other words, when you become fit, you'll know it.

Before you begin the self-assessment phase of your Body Engineering project, there's an important truth to consider. If your renovation efforts are even partially successful, this will be the last time that your body will look or feel as it does now. Recognize that fact and don't become depressed or discouraged if you are less than thrilled with your test results. Radical improvement will occur rapidly as your Body Engineering process unfolds.

Assessment Score Sheet

Test	Points
Home Stress Test	_____
BMR Nocturnal Weight Loss	_____
BMR Waking Temperature	_____
Emotional Stress Test	_____
Flexibility:	
Sit and Reach	_____
Standing Toe Touch	_____
Squat	_____
Torso Twist	_____
Arm Rotations	_____
Ankle Stretch	_____
Strength:	
Push-up	_____
Squat	_____
Crunch	_____
Fast Twitch/Slow Twitch Survey	_____
Jogging Test	_____
Resting Pulse Rate	_____
Body Fat Percentage	_____
TOTAL	_____

Through the Looking Glass and Jump & Jiggle do not have scores but should help you in evaluating the state of your body.

Medical Evaluation

The most accurate method for measuring the current condition of your body's various operating systems is a thorough physical administered by a qualified medical professional. Unfortunately, a comprehensive battery of medical tests is also the least convenient and most expensive evaluation option.

Despite cost considerations, if you are over thirty and have been living a sedentary life for more than three months, consulting a doctor before launching your Body Engineering project is strongly recommended. *If you're a heart patient, a stroke victim, a diabetic, an asthmatic, are afflicted with high blood pressure, or are clinically obese, you absolutely must design your Body Engineering plans under your doctor's supervision.*

Those of you who find the notion of a complete physical impractical or otherwise unappealing should consider submitting to a basic medical exam. A blood analysis and a stress test will tell you most of what you need to know about your internal systems.

Working from blood analyses, your doctor will construct an accurate and useful profile of your current health status. In a professionally administered stress test, a treadmill and a bank of diagnostic monitors measure your body's response to exertion. Electronic analysis of your blood pressure, heart activity, oxygen uptake, and respiration rate as you move through several levels of activity will provide you with an accurate gauge of your current fitness level and capacity for exercise.

The Self-Administered Stress Test

Your everyday activities—from climbing stairs to moving furniture to chasing your kids through the mall—already provide you with a fairly accurate impression of your general fitness level. To

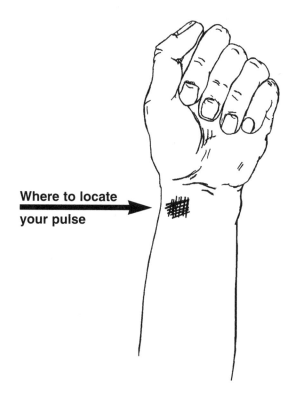

Where to locate your pulse →

quantify this instinctive awareness, you may wish to complete Body Engineering's home version of the stress test.

While the results won't be as precise or as complete as the data available from a professional physiologist, your score in this self-assessment will prove valuable in planning your body renovation process.

To understand your stress test results, you'll need to know how to measure your pulse rate. The best location for your pulse measurements is the radial artery in your wrist. (Although the carotid artery in your neck is easier to find, it often yields inaccurate readings.)

Locate your wrist pulse using the sensitive tips of your index and middle fingers. First, find your wristbone—at the base of your thumb. Then move your fingertips toward your inner wrist. You will feel your pulse in a pocket of flesh. Record the number of pulse beats for one minute. That number is your "resting" pulse rate. The stress test you're going to perform will measure the extent to which exercise affects this rate. Because your pulse rate is an indicator of heart and circulatory system activity, your stress test results will show you the impact of exertion on your body's cardiovascular infrastructure.

Home Stress Test

Important: If your resting pulse rate is over 100, do not take this test.

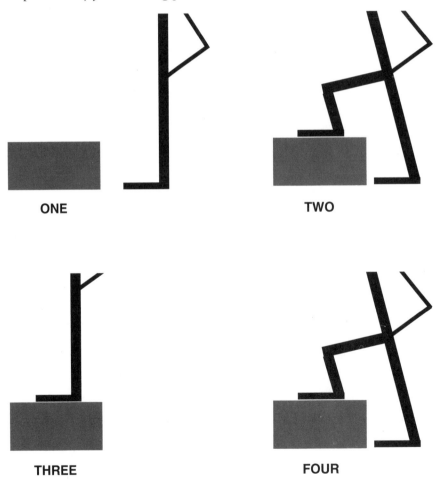

ONE

TWO

THREE

FOUR

The home stress test is fairly simple, but it comes with an important warning: **Stop this test immediately if you experience dizziness, nausea, weakness, chest pain, or extreme shortness of breath. Sit down, recover, and see a doctor as soon as possible.**

1. Find a step, a sturdy box, or a bench 7 or 8 inches high.
2. Measure your pulse rate before starting the test.
3. Start your timer or stopwatch. Climb the step with your left foot. Then bring up your right foot. Both feet are now on the step.
4. Descend with your left foot first, then your right.
5. Continue to climb (left foot), climb (right foot), descend (left foot), descend (right foot) for 1 minute.
6. Count the number of times you bring your left foot up. Try to reach the count of 24 in the 1 minute allotted for the test.
7. When your minute of exertion ends, sit down.
8. Wait 1 minute, then measure your pulse as instructed above. The number of beats per minute (bpm) will determine your general fitness level and your test score.

Under 68 bpm	Excellent: 10 points
68–75 bpm	Good: 5 points
76–80 bpm	Average: 3 points
Over 80 bpm	Below average: 1 point

An average or below average general fitness level can be improved quickly—and significantly—through regular aerobic exercise. A good or excellent fitness level suggests that you are either a physiological marvel or an individual already involved in an active lifestyle.

Basal Metabolic Rate

An important indicator of your body's operational efficiency is your basal metabolic rate (BMR). A comprehensive physical will provide you with an analysis of your metabolism, or you can measure your BMR at home with two simple tests.

BMR Nocturnal Weight Loss

The first **BMR** assessment, while not 100 percent accurate, does offer an adequate approximation of how well your metabolism is working. Simply weigh yourself before you go to sleep at night and again when you wake up in the morning. If a significant weight loss (2 pounds per 100 pounds of body weight) has occurred overnight, your metabolism is working efficiently.

Over 4 lbs. or 3% of body weight	Excellent: 10 points
3–4 lbs. or 2% of body weight	Good: 5 points
1–2 lbs. or 1.5% of body weight	Average: 3 points
Under 1 lb. or 1% of body weight	Below average: 1 point

BMR Waking Temperature

The second test you may wish to use to measure your metabolic rate requires a thermometer rather than a scale. Immediately upon awakening, and while still in bed, place a thermometer under your tongue for ten minutes to record your body temperature. Readings between 97.6 and 98.4 degrees are considered normal. A morning temperature near or exceeding the higher limits of this range suggests that your body is burning calories while you're sleeping—clear evidence of an active, efficient metabolism.

98.6°	Excellent: 10 points
98.2°	Good: 5 points
97.5°	Average: 3 points
Under 97.5°	Below average: 1 point

At regular intervals in your Body Engineering process, use the table below to track your BMR for a week. Record the number of meals you eat, the calories you consume, the duration and intensity of any exercise you perform, and, of course, your weight and temperature readings. At the end of each week, take note of how exercise and eating affect your nocturnal BMR.

BMR Record

Date	Bedtime Weight	Morning Weight	Weight Loss	Waking Temp	Activities	Meals
Ex: 7/23	183 lbs	178 lbs	5 lbs	98.1°	Hard weight training; 40 minutes on bike	5 meals total 2,800 calories

Summary
1. Weigh yourself at bedtime and again in the morning. Record your weight and any net loss.
2. Each morning before you get out of bed, place a thermometer under your tongue for ten minutes and record your temperature.
3. Record activities and meals in order to identify any patterns.

Usually, and certainly not surprisingly, your BMR will be higher on the days you engage in exercise, but it's important to note an exception to that general rule. If you become obsessed with exercise, you may activate a self-defeating cycle. Overexertion, to the point of exhaustion, will lower your BMR dramatically.

Emotional Stress

Emotional stress is a major contributor to a wide array of physical ailments. In fact, stress can be fatal. Stress causes imbalances in all our internal systems, severely disrupting physical and mental harmony and often wreaking bodily harm. If not controlled, stress can silently destroy our most important functional mechanisms.

It is almost impossible to live stress-free in our society (and, frankly, without *some* stress, most of us would wither from boredom); but it *is* possible to learn how to cope effectively with stressful situations. Body Engineering strategies can neutralize the impact of stress on your nervous system, bring order to cerebral chaos, relax the production of fight-or-flight hormones like adrenaline, and avoid depletion of your immune system's essential antibodies.

By learning how best to insulate yourself from predatory stress, you will be arming yourself with a valuable life skill. Your renovation and maintenance strategies must include frequent antistress breaks and an accurate barometer of your current stress levels. Unless you design effective antidotes to eliminate or dilute this harmful toxin, you may become vulnerable to a heart attack or a stroke, or a number of other dangerous ailments.

Emotional Stress Test

I've listed twenty of the most common mental and physical symptoms of stress to assist you in measuring your current level. If you have five or more of the symptoms from the list, you are living with too much stress. If you are experiencing over ten of the stress symptoms listed, seek professional stress-control assistance immediately; your stress level is approaching a dangerous stage.

____ High cholesterol

____ Sexual dysfunction (impotence, lack of interest, etc.)

____ Rapid pulse

____ Loss of appetite

____ Nausea

____ Stomach queasiness ("butterflies")

____ Heartburn

____ Stiff neck

____ Sweaty palms

____ Frequent headaches

____ Insomnia

____ Fatigue

____ High blood pressure

____ Binge eating

____ Teeth grinding

____ Chronic diarrhea or constipation

____ General anxiety

____ Irritability

____ Can't sit still

____ Indecisiveness

0–1 symptom	Excellent: 10 points
2–3 symptoms	Good: 5 points
4–5 symptoms	Average: 3 points
6 or more symptoms	Below average: 1 point

Adapted from ISSA.

Fitness Factors

Fitness is sometimes described in terms of the following attributes: strength, endurance, agility, speed, coordination, flexibility, balance, muscle control, low levels of body fat, and high levels of energy. However, the interrelation of all the components of overall fitness makes fitness difficult to accurately measure.

Unlike tests for blood pressure and heart rate, there are no universally recognized standard measures for all the elements that define fitness. However, the Body Engineering process helps you to establish your own personal fitness standards. Instead of being overly concerned with inches and pounds and recovery times, concentrate on determining the level of fitness you need to enjoy the kind of life you want to live.

Fitness is not a single ideal physical state. An infinite variety of goals, needs, and lifestyles requires an infinite variety of radically different levels of fitness and body development standards. While it's safe to say that in some measure strength, endurance, and flexibility are essential aspects of fitness, one or another of these elements may be more or less vital to any one individual, depending on his or her age, activities preferences, family responsibilities, career demands, and so forth.

Fortunately, engineering is a subjective, practical discipline that recognizes that there are often at least several viable solutions to any given problem. Employing as much life experience and art as mathematics and physics, the best engineers rely on intuition and sensory input to blend the ideal with the realistic.

As you work through Body Engineering's process, you'll discover that many features of the new body you're striving to create can't be defined by a set of measurements, or even by verbal descriptions. While numbers on a chart will be useful, you are likely to find yourself much more interested in how your evolving body looks and feels and moves.

In deference to the unique definition of fitness that each body engineer will develop individually and independently, assessment exercises measuring flexibility, endurance and strength focus exclusively on basics—general fitness factors that will be present to some extent regardless of your specific fitness goals.

FLEXIBILITY

Any exercise strategy you ultimately devise will require some degree of flexibility. Cold muscles and stiff joints are susceptible to injury and incapable of optimum performance. While you need not achieve a high level of flexibility to exercise, a supple physique will certainly expand the scope of your workout options and increase your enjoyment of recreational activities.

The flexibility test that follows consists of six exercises designed to determine muscle and joint mobility and range of motion. Carefully follow the instructions and record your results after completing each movement. Be cautious as you proceed. Stretch slowly and patiently. Don't force movement if your body protests.

These exercises are useful for warming up before workouts and cooling down afterward. Because flexibility movements of some sort will become an important part of your exercise routine, concentrate on completing these test exercises correctly. Again, move slowly and carefully and *stop immediately if you feel any strain.*

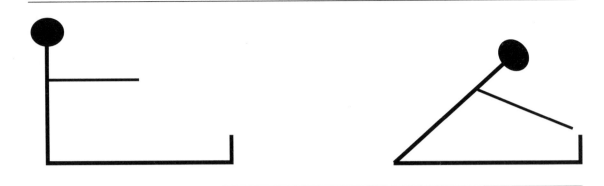

Sit and Reach

While seated on the floor, bring your feet together and lock your knees. Extend your arms, reach forward, and attempt to touch your toes. Bending and reaching as far as you can without discomfort, hold this position for 7 to 10 seconds. Don't bounce or rock, simply stretch. Release slowly, relax for 10 seconds, then repeat the Sit and Reach at least 2 more times. How close you can come to your toes during this stretch provides an indication of the range of motion of your lower back and hamstrings.

Reach past toes	Excellent: 10 points
Reach to toes	Good: 5 points
Reach to top of feet	Average: 3 points
Touch ankles	Below average: 1 point

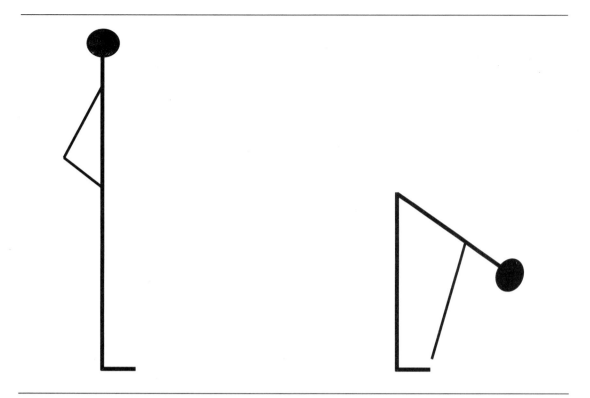

Standing Toe Touch

Stand with your knees locked and your feet spread no wider than the width of your shoulders. Slowly lower your upper body by bending at the waistline. Try to touch your toes, or the floor, but don't strain to do so. Bend slowly and steadily until your body tells you to stop. Hold this position for 7 to 10 seconds, relax, and repeat at least 2 more times. How far you can bend will indicate the range of motion in your lower back, upper legs, and calves.

Palms touch floor	Excellent: 10 points
Fingers touch toes	Good: 5 points
Fingers touch top of feet	Average: 3 points
Fingers touch ankles	Below average: 1 point

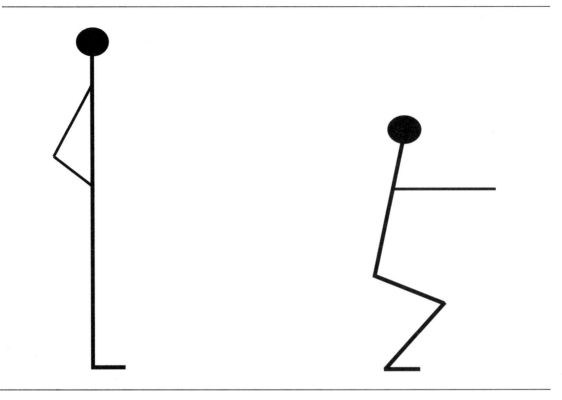

Squat

Stand upright with your feet flat on the floor and spaced slightly wider than shoulder width. With your toes pointed outward just a bit, bend your knees and ankles, squatting down slowly until your heels start to leave the floor. Pause at this point for 2 to 5 seconds, then slowly return to the upright position. Repeat 3 to 5 times. When you become comfortable in the squat position, you can rock slightly from side to side to loosen up the knees, ankles, hips, and surrounding muscles.

Hamstrings touch calf	Excellent: 10 points
Thighs below parallel	Good: 5 points
Thighs parallel	Average: 3 points
Thighs above parallel	Below average: 1 point

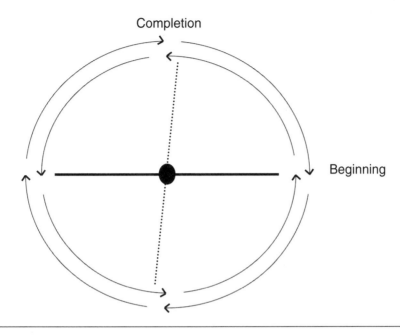

Top View

Completion

Beginning

Torso Twist

While standing with feet just wider than shoulder width apart, extend your arms straight out to the side until they are parallel to the floor. Lock your upper body and arms and pivot as far as possible, first to the left, then to the right. Move your entire upper body, not merely your arms and shoulders. After pivoting slowly as far as you can to one side, hold your position for 7 to 10 seconds. Release slowly and rotate to the other side. When you have reached full rotation, hold for 7 to 10 seconds. Perform 2 or 3 full rotations to each side. The object of this movement is to determine range of motion in your lower back and abdominal girdle.

Left or right arm crosses
    opposite foot   Excellent: 10 points
Arm reaches past 90°   Good: 5 points
Arm reaches between feet (90°)   Average: 3 points
Arm reaches less than 90°   Below average: 1 point

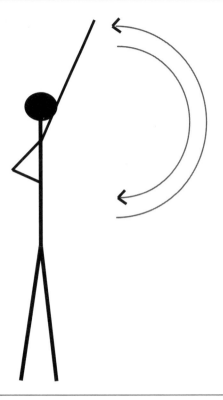

Arm Rotations

Lock your right elbow and lift your right arm to shoulder level and extend it in front of you. Bring your arm up in an arc, as high overhead as possible, and as far behind you as your range of motion will allow. Repeat the movement with your left arm. Alternate between arms, performing a minimum of 5 rotations with each. Always perform this movement slowly, reaching as far in front, as high, and as far behind as you can. The object is to make the largest circle possible. The size of the arc you can inscribe indicates the range of motion of your shoulder joints and muscles, the pectorals, upper back, and triceps.

Large, tight circle	Excellent: 10 points
Large, wide circle	Good: 5 points
Medium, wide circle	Average: 3 points
Small, wide circle	Below average: 1 point

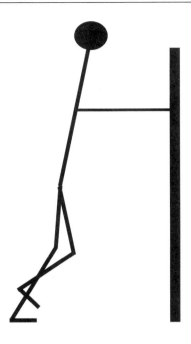

Ankle Stretch

Place both hands on a wall at chest height. Keeping your right heel on the floor, step forward with your left leg. This lunge will stretch your right ankle, calf, and Achilles tendon. Hold the deepest stretch you can for 7 to 10 seconds. Release slowly, switch legs, and stretch again. Alternate between legs at least 3 times. Try to bend the ankle as much as possible without strain or discomfort.

Knee 3 or more inches past toes	Excellent: 10 points
Knee 1 inch past toes	Good: 5 points
Knee at toes	Average: 3 points
Knee behind toes	Below average: 1 point

STRENGTH

In engineering terms, strength is a measure of structural integrity. An engineering team formulating the design of a mechanical apparatus of any sort needs to know the level of force each component of the new machine will exert and the amount of stress each moving part can bear.

The body engineer faces similar concerns. The body's muscles are the source of all physical movement, and a reasonable level of strength is critical to the success of all fitness strategies.

The personal strength tests that follow will provide an accurate assessment of your current strength level. Keep in mind that strength is an aspect of fitness that you can improve almost immediately. Well-planned, conscientiously executed resistance training typically produces noticeable strength gains within one week.

Complete as many repetitions as possible for each of the following exercises. Record your scores.

Push-Up

Lie facedown and place your hands underneath your shoulders, adjacent to your chest. While keeping your body rigid, push yourself up until your arms lock. Now lower yourself slowly until your chest slightly contacts the floor. Repeat.

20+	Excellent: 10 points
12–19	Good: 5 points
5–11	Average: 3 points
0–4	Below average: 1 point

Squat

Stand upright with your feet a little more than shoulder width apart, toes slightly pointed outward. Keeping your back straight, bend at your hips and knees to lower yourself until your thighs are parallel to the floor. Push upward until your legs straighten. Repeat.

25+	Excellent: 10 points
15–24	Good: 5 points
10–14	Average: 3 points
0–9	Below average: 1 point

Crunch

Lie faceup with your hands resting on your upper abdominals. Bend your knees until your feet are flat against the floor. Lift your upper back 2 to 3 inches from the floor and hold for a count of 3. Lower and repeat.

30+	Excellent: 10 points
20–29	Good: 5 points
10–19	Average: 3 points
0–9	Below average: 1 point

Muscle Fibers

Muscle fibers—single narrow cells running the entire length of each muscle—are the basic unit of physical activity. Thousands of these fibers contract powerfully and in unison when a muscle is activated.

Human muscle is comprised of two distinct fiber types. *Fast twitch* (FT) fibers are thick, but house only a few blood vessels. FT fibers contract explosively and forcefully. These are the body tissues that enable you to spike a volleyball, lift weights, sprint, and leap (fast twitch = fast movement). FT fibers are extremely powerful, but they tire quickly because they exhaust available energy resources so rapidly. (FT energy supplies are derived primarily from carbohydrates.)

Slow twitch (ST) fibers are laced with blood vessels. Their abundant energy sources are activated when we walk, jog, or engage in any steadily paced aerobic activity (slow twitch = slow movement). ST fibers are less powerful than FT fibers but far superior in endurance. (The main energy sources for ST fibers are oxygen, carbohydrates, and fat.)

For example, Joe sprints full tilt for one hundred yards. At the finish line, Joe finds it difficult to speak because he is gasping for oxygen. His internal systems are busy increasing respiration to replenish the energy he has expended so suddenly.

A moment after Joe's sprint ends, Joan walks the same hundred yards. She crosses the finish line and keeps on going. Joan has no trouble carrying on an animated conversation, or singing show tunes, for that matter. If Joan wants to, she can walk and talk at this pace for hours.

Fast twitch muscle fibers made Joe's sprint possible, while slow twitch fibers facilitated Joan's stroll. Each fiber type performed its function using different metabolic pathways and different fuel sources.

Each of us is born with a genetically controlled percentage of FT and ST fibers in relation to our lean-muscle mass, and usually these ratios do not change as we age. An individual with a high volume of ST fibers will tend to excel in activities like cross-country skiing and long-distance running, while someone with a high FT fiber percentage can probably become a successful sprinter, boxer, or gymnast. There are, of course, thousands of exceptions to this general rule. Mental skills, sheer desire, and unique coordination factors often give certain athletes the ability to overcome genetic "handicaps" and excel at sports that they're not really "built" for.

There is also a third type of muscle matter—*FST fibers*, a combination of FT and ST elements. FST is a convertible fiber that we can modify for specific purposes. If you train for aerobic activities, you are training your FST fibers to act and react like slow twitch fibers. On the other hand, training for quick, explosive activities like basketball or heavy weight lifting will "teach" certain FST fibers to behave like fast twitch fibers.

It is possible to convert and reengineer enough muscle fibers so that you are not restricted to any single type of exercise. This capability offers obvious advantages for those of you who want to maximize performance in a variety of dissimilar recreational or competitive activities.

Fast Twitch/Slow Twitch Survey

This self-assessment will help you determine whether your body is FT- or ST-oriented. Knowing your predominant muscle fiber type will be valuable later as you design specific elements of your Body Engineering process. Keep in mind, however, that many activities require a combination of muscle fibers.

In the survey below, put a checkmark next to the entry that best describes yourself.

I am more prone to:	__Walking, jogging	__Running, sprinting
I consider my muscles:	__Not strong enough	__Strong
My energy levels are:	__Low to okay	__High
I am more apt to play sports like:	__Golf or pool	__Basketball, tennis, racquetball
I enjoy lifting heavy weights:	__No, not really	__Yes
I am able to jump:	__Not at all; not very high	__Very well
I can throw a ball:	__Not too far	__Very far
I eat a lot but don't get fat:	__Not me	__Yes

---

5 or more on the right-
   hand column   Excellent: 10 points
4 on both columns   Good: 5 points
5 on the left column   Average: 3 points
6–8 on the left column   Below average: 1 point

CARDIORESPIRATORY ENDURANCE

Testing endurance (a fitness factor often referred to as aerobic capacity) is relatively easy, and for some novice body engineers, not really necessary. If you find yourself short of breath after performing even moderately taxing physical activities, you already know that you need to improve this aspect of fitness.

Almost all of us possess sufficient endurance to live a sedentary life. But if you want to get out into the world and try something physically challenging (and/or fun), reengineering your body's cardiorespiratory system will be necessary.

Endurance is a function of your body's ability to process oxygen. Endurance deficiencies arise when our cardiovascular and respiratory systems are unable to convert oxygen into usable fuel for the kinetic energy we need to sustain physical activity. As you will discover in the initial phases of the engineering process, a regular schedule of low-impact aerobic exercise can dramatically increase the stamina and proficiency of your heart and lungs in less than an hour a day. Beneficial results of the endurance boosters you may choose to incorporate into your renovation plans should become apparent about three weeks into the process.

Jogging Test

A number of endurance tests are frequently prescribed by trainers and cardiologists. Perhaps the simplest involves jogging.

After a 10-to-15 minute warm-up (the flexibility test exercises are an excellent way to begin), jog for as long as you can without discomfort. When your body tells you that it's time to stop, stop. **Note: Don't push yourself. Stop immediately if you experience dizziness, nausea, weakness, chest pain, or extreme shortness of breath. Sit down, recover, and see a doctor as soon as possible.**

Compare the length of time you were able to jog with the standards listed at the top of page 97 for an approximate but adequate estimate of your current endurance level.

Heart Rate

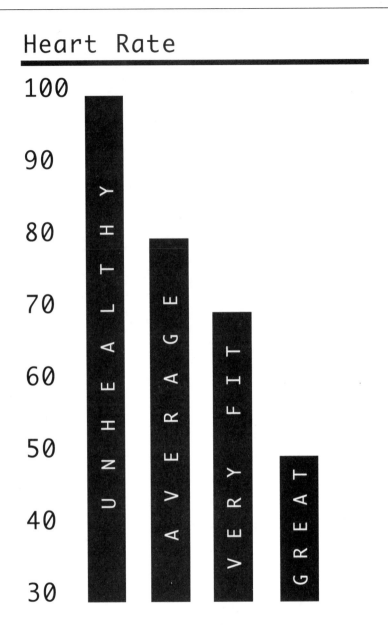

45–60 minutes	Excellent: 10 points
30–44 minutes	Good: 5 points
20–29 minutes	Average: 3 points
1–19 minutes	Below average: 1 point

CARDIOVASCULAR EFFICIENCY

An efficient heart will pump more blood with each beat than an unfit heart; so the lower your heartbeat, the more efficient your heart is. Some top athletes have resting heart rates below 50 beats per minute. In contrast, an unfit person's heart rate may be well above 80.

Resting Pulse Rate

Check your pulse right now and then use the chart on page 96 to estimate your cardiovascular efficiency.

Under 60 bpm	Excellent: 10 points
61–70 bpm	Good: 5 points
71–80 bpm	Average: 3 points
Over 80 bpm	Below average: 1 point

Body Measurements

Several reliable measurement devices are available to evaluate body composition and lean-tissue levels. Your bathroom scale isn't one of them.

As you work through your Body Engineering process, there will be periods of time when your weight seems stubbornly immune to your exercise and eating strategies. Don't worry about it. Scales are inaccurate and misleading progress indicators. Muscle by volume is heavier than fat, but muscle occupies less than one-third the body mass that fat displaces.

Body Measurement Progress Chart

DATE								
Height								
Weight								
Neck								
Shoulders								
Chest								
Bust								
Waist								
Hips								
Thigh (R)								
Thigh (L)								
Knee (R)								
Knee (L)								
Calf (R)								
Calf (L)								
Ankle (R)								
Ankle (L)								
Biceps (R)								
Biceps (L)								
Forearm (R)								
Forearm (L)								
Wrist (R)								
Wrist (L)								

Comparing your current body measurements to those you'll collect later in your renovation process will provide convincing (and valid) evidence that progress in reshaping and reproportioning your body is indeed being made.

To assemble your baseline body composition data, measure each of the body areas indicated in the assessment chart on page 98. As you perform these measurements, be careful not to compress skin or flesh. Record your current measurements for future reference. Every ten to fifteen days during your Body Engineering process, re-measure to track your progress.

Body Fat

The United States is one of the fattest nations in the world—which explains why most health and fitness novices are motivated by the desire to become lighter and leaner.

Excess fat interferes with several of the body's essential functions and is the primary cause of most heart disease. Reaching and maintaining an acceptable body fat level is a basic element of your Body Engineering process.

Knowing your body fat percentage—that is, what percentage of your body tissue is fat—will help you to quantify your fat-reduction goals, and, as your Body Engineering process evolves, provide a convenient benchmark for determining exactly where you are in relation to those goals.

Most of the commonly used tests that claim to calculate body fat percentage, however, are error prone and extremely expensive. Inaccuracies occur because of the influences of intramuscular fat levels, intestinal waste, gut gases, and body hydration. Even though these "scientific" tests don't correctly assess body fat levels, clinics and trainers around the country continue to use them—because it's profitable to do so.

Body Fat Percentage

There's no need to waste your time and money to determine your body fat level. The following test costs nothing and is easily administered at home.

WOMEN

---

1. Determine standing height (without shoes) in inches.
2. Measure hip girth at the widest point in inches.
3. Using the chart below, draw a straight line from hip girth measurement (on the left) to standing height (on the right).
4. Find the point where the line crosses the middle scale. This is your estimated body fat percentage.

For example, a woman with a hip girth of 36 inches who is 60 inches (5 feet) tall has an estimated 26 percent of fat (determined by drawing a line from 36 on the left to 60 on the right and finding that the line crosses the percent fat at 26).

Calculating Body Fat Percentages: Women

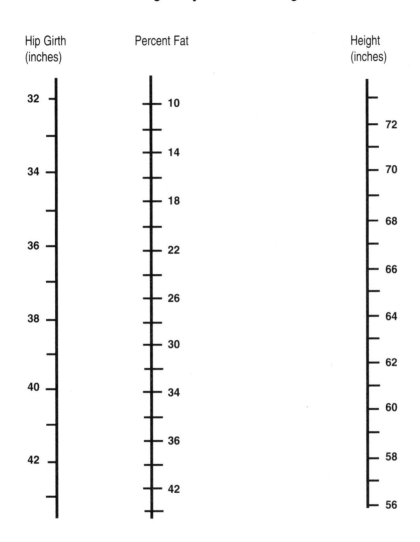

This chart estimates relative fat percentages in women based on hip girth and height. Adapted from Wilmore (1986).

Calculating Body Fat Percentages: Men

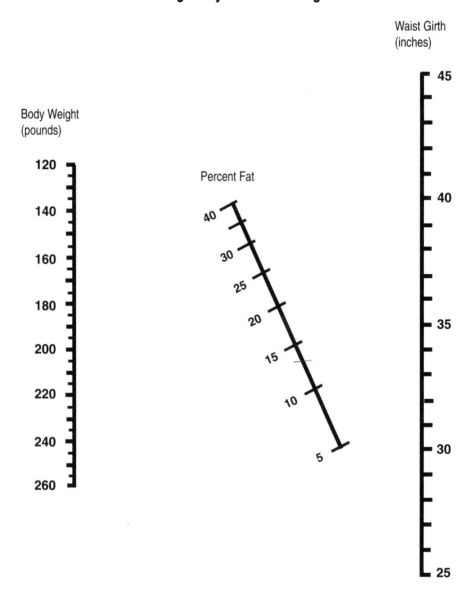

This chart estimates relative fat percentages in men based on body weight and abdominal or waistline circumference.
Adapted from Wilmore (1986).

1. Determine weight in pounds.
2. Measure waist girth at the widest point in inches.
3. Using the chart below, draw a straight line from body weight (on the left) to waist girth (on the right).
4. Find the point where the line crosses the middle section. This is your estimated body fat percentage.

For example, a man who weighs 200 pounds with a waist girth of 40 inches has an estimated 26 percent of fat.

Curious about how you rank in comparison to objective body composition standards?

MEN

Under 9%	Excellent: 10 points
9–12%	Good: 5 points
13–19%	Average: 3 points
20% or more	Below average: 1 point

WOMEN

Under 15%	Excellent: 10 points
15–22%	Good: 5 points
23–29%	Average: 3 points
30% or more	Below average: 1 point

Before your new body can exist in the physical world, it must emerge as an image, an idea, a mental picture, a glimpse of potential.

Despite its technical underpinnings, engineering is a visual, intuitive, nonverbal discipline. Successful design efforts combine formal knowledge with sensory experience, and, almost always, the engineering process relies more on subjective judgment than objective certainty. All of which explains why your final assessment exercise isn't the least bit scientific.

THROUGH THE LOOKING GLASS

Many features of your new body can't be charted or measured or weighed. To sharpen the focus of your renovation plan, your mind requires sensory images. The same "imaging" techniques that skilled engineers employ to set design goals and to create detailed drawings of structures that will not be built for years can be a valuable aid in finalizing your self-improvement project plan.

You can use photos or role models to help you visualize what your new body will look like, or you can use a mirror to provide you with a preview of the future.

Stand before a full-length mirror that permits you to view your entire body (front, sides, and rear). After bringing yourself as close to naked as you can stand, exhale while flexing your muscles. Expand your chest and tighten your abdominals.

What you will see gazing back at you is a life-size representation of the body that awaits you at some point in your Body Engineering process. Depending on your current physical condition, this image may be hazy and incomplete and less than satisfactory, or it may be crystal-clear and quite pleasing. In either case, you will have shown yourself a valuable projection of what lies ahead—useful, at the very least, in establishing a reasonable intermediate goal.

Jump and Jiggle

Since you're dressed for it anyway, you may wish to conclude your time before the mirror with one more visual aid—a goofy-looking but possibly helpful evaluation exercise I call the Jump and Jiggle test.

Flex your muscles. Then, using short rapid bounces, jump up and down. You need to bounce only high enough to bring both feet off the floor. As you bounce, telltale jiggling will pinpoint body areas where excess fat has accumulated. This information helps you select toning exercises that will isolate these problem sites and will eventually allow you to see how your exercise strategies are reshaping your entire physique.

Repeat this evaluation technique every two weeks during your renovation effort. Be a dispassionate self-critic, objective and honest about what you see. As you work your way through your Body Engineering project, don't be surprised if your critiques become more and more positive.

CHAPTER FIVE

Product Design

Four Templates to Help You Build Your New Body with Nutrition and Exercise

A template, as many of you home computer owners know, is an information "stencil" used to create reports, business plans, budgets, mailing lists, and spreadsheets.

The template's structure "prompts" the software user for the type, class, or category of information needed to produce a finished document. The user simply enters data unique to the project's requirements.

User-friendly templates are fluid organizational aids, easily modified or fine-tuned at the user's discretion. The Body Engineering templates presented in this chapter are based on well-established, thoroughly tested health and fitness principles. Each template is designed to serve as a foundational guide for a nutrition and activity plan you can customize to meet your individual needs, desires, and goals.

The self-assessment tests you completed in chapter 4 helped you to evaluate your current physical condition. Begin with these findings to choose the appropriate template. If your total assessment score was in the range of 160–180, you should probably select the Sports Performance template. The Health Maintenance template is the likely choice for people with a score of 90–159. The Weight Loss or Weight Gain template will be right for people with scores of 18–89. But remember that *the way you look and feel* is ultimately the most accurate way to select the right template.

Do the assessments every 6 to 8 weeks to collect up-to-date baseline data. You may switch to an alternative template as your progress dictates.

Please note that each Body Engineering template includes separate nutrition and exercise components.

Template 1 (Weight Loss) will be the starting point for most new body engineers. This template's guidelines are designed to improve overall fitness, build functional strength, recharge metabolism, and burn fat.

Template 2 (Weight Gain) shows how body engineers seeking size and strength improvements can build muscle power and mass.

Template 3 (Health Maintenance) will be a valuable aid to body engineers who are presently fit and who want to stay that way.

Template 4 (Sports Performance) offers high-intensity workout plans and nutritional advice for athletes at all levels of physical competition.

TEMPLATE 1. WEIGHT LOSS

Weight Loss Nutrition: Choose items from the Nutritional Menu (pages 122–125). Select one or two fats daily. Use supplements as appropriate. (Serving size is 1 unless otherwise noted in parentheses.)

	OPTION 1	OPTION 2
MEAL 1 6–10 A.M.	Carb-Simple (2) _____ Protein _____ Beverage _____	Carb-Starch _____ Carb-Simple (2)_____ Beverage _____
SNACK 2 hours after first meal	Carb-Simple (2)_____ Beverage_____	Carb-Fibrous (2) _____ Beverage _____
MEAL 2 Noon–2 P.M.	Protein_____ Carb-Fibrous (2)_____ Beverage_____	Protein_____ Carb-Simple _____ Carb-Fibrous _____ Beverage_____
MEAL 3 4–7 P.M.	Carb-Starch_____ Carb-Fibrous (2)_____ Protein_____ Beverage_____	Protein_____ Carb-Fibrous (2)_____ Beverage _____
SNACK 2 hours after last meal or 2 hours before bedtime	Carb-Fibrous (3)_____ Beverage_____	Carb-Starch _____ Carb-Fibrous (2)_____ Beverage _____

Weight Loss Fitness

MONDAY	TUESDAY	WEDNESDAY	THURSDAY	FRIDAY	SATURDAY	SUNDAY
Strength Workout 1	No Strength	Strength Workout 2	Rest	Strength Workout 1	No Strength	Rest
Aerobics 20–40 minutes	Aerobics 30–60 minutes	Aerobics 20–40 minutes		Aerobics 30–60 minutes	Aerobics 30–60 minutes	

Strength Workout

WORKOUT 1	WORKOUT 2
Choose one exercise per line.	Choose one exercise per line.
Muscle	**Muscle**
Total body _____	Total body _____
Chest _____	Legs _____
Legs _____	Upper abs _____
Shoulders _____	Lower abs _____
Hips _____	Buttocks _____
Biceps _____	Triceps _____
Upper abs _____	Inner thighs _____
Upper back _____	Shoulders _____
Hamstrings _____	Calves _____
Obliques _____	Lower back _____

Instructions

Always complete your strength routine first.

Strength

- Begin with the flexibility test exercises from chapter 4.
- Choose a strength activity for each muscle group from the Anaerobic Exercise Menu (page 130).
- All exercises will be conducted for 2 or 3 sets.
     Upper body exercises: 12–25 reps
     Lower body exercises: 15–30 reps
- Do not rest more than 30 seconds between sets.

Aerobic

- Choose an activity from the Aerobic Exercise Menu (page 129).
- Perform at 70–80 percent of your target heart rate. **Formula:** 220 minus your age multiplied by 70–80 percent equals your target heart rate.
     Ex: $220 - 32 = 188 \times 80\% = 150$.
     150 is your maximum target heart rate.
- Cool down with the flexibility test exercises from chapter 4.

TEMPLATE 2. WEIGHT GAIN

Weight Gain Nutrition: Choose items from the Nutritional Menu (pages 122–125). Select three or four fats daily. Use supplements as appropriate. (Serving size is 1 unless otherwise noted in parentheses.)

	OPTION 1	OPTION 2
MEAL 1 6–10 A.M.	Protein (2) _____ Carb-Starch (3) _____ Carb-Simple (2) _____ Beverage _____	Protein (2) _____ Carb-Starch (2) _____ Carb-Fibrous (2) _____ Beverage _____
SNACK 2 hours after first meal	Carb-Simple (2) _____ Beverage _____	Carb-Fibrous (2) _____ Protein (2) _____ Beverage _____
MEAL 2 Noon–2 P.M.	Protein (2) _____ Carb-Fibrous (3) _____ Carb-Starch (2) _____ Beverage_____	Protein (2) _____ Carb-Starch (2) _____ Carb-Fibrous (3) _____ Beverage _____
MEAL 3 3–6 P.M.	Protein (2) _____ Carb-Starch (3) _____ Carb-Simple (2) _____ Beverage _____	Protein (2) _____ Carb-Starch (2) _____ Carb-Fibrous (2) _____ Beverage _____

MEAL 4 6–9 P.M.	Protein (2) _____ Carb-Fibrous (2) _____ Carb-Starch (2) _____ Beverage _____	Protein (2) _____ Carb-Starch (2) _____ Carb-Fibrous (3) _____ Beverage _____
SNACK 2 hours after last meal or 1 hour before bedtime	Carb-Starch (2) _____ Protein _____ Beverage—————————	Protein (2) _____ Carb-Fibrous _____ Carb-Starch _____ Beverage _____

Weight Gain Fitness

MONDAY	TUESDAY	WEDNESDAY	THURSDAY	FRIDAY	SATURDAY	SUNDAY
Strength Workout 1	**Strength** Workout 2	**No Strength**	**Strength** Workout 3	**No Strength**	**Strength** Workout 1	**Rest**
Aerobics 20 minutes	**No Aerobics**	**Aerobics** 20–30 minutes	**No Aerobics**	**Aerobics** 20–30 minutes	**Aerobics** 20 minutes	

Strength Workout

WORKOUT 1	WORKOUT 2	WORKOUT 3

Choose one exercise per line.

Muscle

Chest _____

Chest _____

Chest _____

Upper back _____

Upper back _____

Biceps _____

Biceps _____

Choose one exercise per line.

Muscle

Total body _____

Legs _____

Legs _____

Hamstrings _____

Calves _____

Lower back _____

Upper abs _____

Lower abs _____

Obliques _____

Choose one exercise per line.

Muscle

Total body _____

Shoulders _____

Shoulders _____

Shoulders _____

Triceps _____

Triceps _____

Instructions

Always complete your strength routine first.

Strength
- Begin with the flexibility test exercises from chapter 4.
- Choose a strength activity for each muscle group from the Anaerobic Exercise Menu (page 130).
- All exercises will be conducted for 3 or 4 sets.
    Upper body exercises: 6–15 reps
    Lower body exercises: 8–20 reps

Aerobic
- Choose an activity from the Aerobic Exercise Menu (page 129).
- Perform at 60–90 percent of your target heart rate. **Formula:** 220 minus your age multiplied by 60–90 percent equals your target heart rate.
    Ex: $220 - 32 = 188 \times 90\% = 169$.
    169 is your maximum target heart rate.
- Cool down with the flexibility test exercises from chapter 4.

TEMPLATE 3. HEALTH MAINTENANCE

Health Maintenance Nutrition: Choose items from the Nutritional Menu (pages 122–125). Select two or three fats daily. Use supplements as appropriate. (Serving size is 1 unless otherwise noted in parentheses.)

	OPTION 1	OPTION 2
MEAL 1 6–10 A.M.	Carb-Simple (2) _____ Beverage _____	Protein _____ Carb-Starch _____ Carb-Simple _____ Beverage_____
SNACK 2 hours after first meal	Carb-Simple (2) _____ Beverage _____	Carb-Fibrous (2) _____ Beverage _____
MEAL 2 Noon–2 P.M.	Protein_____ Carb-Fibrous (2)_____ Beverage_____	Protein _____ Carb-Simple _____ Carb-Fibrous (2) _____ Beverage _____
MEAL 3 4–7 P.M.	Protein _____ Carb-Starch _____ Carb-Fibrous _____ Beverage _____	Protein _____ Carb-Fibrous (2) _____ Beverage _____
SNACK 2 hours after last meal or 2 hours before bedtime	Carb-Fibrous (3) _____ Beverage _____	Carb-Starch _____ Carb-Fibrous (2) _____ Beverage _____

Health Maintenance Fitness

MONDAY	TUESDAY	WEDNESDAY	THURSDAY	FRIDAY	SATURDAY	SUNDAY
Strength Workout 1	No Strength	Strength Workout 2	Rest	No Strength	Strength Workout 1	Rest
Aerobics 15–30 minutes	Aerobics 20–45 minutes	Aerobics 15–30 minutes		Aerobics 30–60 minutes	No Aerobics	

Strength Workout

WORKOUT 1	WORKOUT 2

Choose one exercise per line.

Muscle

Total body _____

Shoulders _____

Legs _____

Chest _____

Hips _____

Upper back _____

Upper abs _____

Triceps _____

Hamstrings _____

Obliques _____

Choose one exercise per line.

Muscle

Total body _____

Lower back _____

Upper abs _____

Legs _____

Buttocks _____

Biceps _____

Inner thighs _____

Shoulders _____

Lower abs _____

Calves _____

Instructions

Always complete your strength routine first.

Strength
- Begin with the flexibility test exercises from chapter 4.
- Choose a strength activity for each muscle group from the Anaerobic Exercise Menu (page 130).
- All exercises will be conducted for 3 or 4 sets.
    Upper body exercises: 10–15 reps
    Lower body exercises: 12–20 reps
- Rest no longer than 30 seconds between sets.

Aerobic
- Choose an activity from the Aerobic Exercise Menu (page 129).
- Perform at 60–85 percent of your target heart rate. **Formula:** 220 minus your age multiplied by 60–85 percent equals your target heart rate.
    Ex: 220 − 32 = 188 × 85% = 160.
    160 is your maximum target heart rate.
- Cool down with the flexibility test exercises from chapter 4.

TEMPLATE 4. SPORTS PERFORMANCE

Sports Performance Nutrition: Choose items from the Nutritional Menu (pages 122–125). Select three or four fats daily. Use supplements as appropriate. (Serving size is 1 unless otherwise noted in parentheses.)

	OPTION 1	OPTION 2
MEAL 1 6–10 A.M.	Protein (2) _____ Carb-Starch (3) _____ Carb-Simple (2) _____ Beverage _____	Protein (2)_____ Carb-Starch (2) _____ Carb-Fibrous (2)_____ Carb-Simple (2)_____ Beverage_____
SNACK 2 hours after first meal	Carb-Simple (2)_____ Beverage_____	Carb-Starch (2) _____ Protein (2)_____ Beverage _____
MEAL 2 Noon–2 P.M.	Protein (2) _____ Carb-Fibrous (2)_____ Carb-Starch (3)_____ Beverage_____	Protein (2) _____ Carb-Starch (2) _____ Carb-Fibrous (2)_____ Carb-Simple_____ Beverage _____
MEAL 3 3–5 P.M.	Protein (2) _____ Carb-Starch (3) _____ Carb-Simple (2) _____ Beverage _____	Protein (2)_____ Carb-Starch (2) _____ Carb-Fibrous (3)_____ Beverage_____

MEAL 4 6–9 P.M.	Protein (2) _____ Carb-Fibrous (3)_____ Carb-Starch (2)_____ Beverage _____	Protein (2)_____ Carb-Starch (2) _____ Carb-Fibrous (3)_____ Beverage_____
SNACK 1–2 hours after last meal or 1 hour before bedtime	Carb-Starch (2) _____ Protein _____ Beverage _____	Protein (2) _____ Carb-Fibrous _____ Carb-Starch _____ Beverage_____

Sports Performance Fitness

MONDAY	TUESDAY	WEDNESDAY	THURSDAY	FRIDAY	SATURDAY	SUNDAY
Strength Workout 1	Strength Workout 2	No Strength	Rest	Strength Workout 3	Strength Workout 1	Rest
Aerobics 20–30 minutes	Aerobics 20–45 minutes	Aerobics 20–30 minutes		Aerobics 20–45 minutes	Aerobics 40–60 minutes	

Strength Workout

WORKOUT 1	WORKOUT 2	WORKOUT 3
Choose one exercise per line.	Choose one exercise per line.	Choose one exercise per line.
Muscle	**Muscle**	**Muscle**
Chest _____	Total body_____	Total body_____
Chest _____	Legs _____	Shoulders _____
Chest _____	Legs _____	Shoulders _____
Upper back _____	Legs _____	Shoulders _____
Upper back _____	Legs _____	Shoulders _____
Triceps_____	Hamstrings _____	Biceps _____
Triceps_____	Calves _____	Biceps _____
	Lower back _____	Obliques _____
	Upper abs_____	Lower abs_____

Instructions

Always complete your strength routine first.

Strength
- Begin with the flexibility test exercises from chapter 4.
- Choose a strength activity for each muscle group from the Anaerobic Exercise Menu (page 130).
- All exercises will be conducted for 3 or 4 sets.
  Upper body exercises: 6–12 reps
  Lower body exercises: 8–15 reps

Aerobic
- Choose an activity from the Aerobic Exercise Menu (page 129).
- Perform at 75–95 percent of your target heart rate. **Formula:** 220 minus your age multiplied by 75–95 percent equals your target heart rate.
  Ex: $220 - 32 = 188 \times 95\% = 179$.
  179 is your maximum target heart rate.
- Cool down with the flexibility test exercises from chapter 4.

Nutrition

The nutrition component of each Body Engineering template indicates the types of food most compatible with your weight, body composition, and functionality goals. The *specific* foods you consume and the natural supplements you add to your eating plan are entirely up to you. Eat a variety of foods and don't hesitate to try new dishes or exotic combinations of foods you like. If you succumb to an occasional Big Mac Attack or fall victim to Donut Dementia, don't agonize over it. Just be sure to make better meal choices the next time. Don't give up after a little slip. Prolong or intensify your next workout to bring yourself back on track. If your lifestyle forces you to rely on prepackaged meals to any degree, remember to read labels carefully. Limit high-fat and high-sugar items and avoid products that seem more chemical than organic. Don't forget:

- Eat reasonably sized meals several times a day.
- Don't deny yourself any food you crave; make room for these necessary pleasures in your eating plan.
- Choose fresh foods over processed products, but if your life is too complex or fast-paced to allow for thoughtful meal preparation, be sure to read the labels of the dozens of frozen entrées now offered by Healthy Choice, Lean Cuisine, Weight Watchers, et al. Several of these products are at least adequate, and some are excellent. All are portion controlled, with calories and fat grams already counted for you.
- Don't rush through meals—relax and enjoy your food. Eat slowly. Experience the food's texture, aroma, and taste.
- Drink lots of water.
- Think of food as fuel, not as an escape, a reward, or a friend.
- Visit a health or nutrition professional for assistance in designing an appropriate supplement plan.

Nutritional Menu

Protein	1 Serving
Eggs	2 (2 whites, 1 yolk)
Turkey	8 oz.
Ham	8 oz.
Chicken	8 oz.
Meat (lean red)	8 oz.
Fish	8 oz.
Jumbo shrimp	4
Cheese (low- or no-fat)	2 oz.
Cottage cheese (low-fat, low-sodium)	4 oz.

Carbohydrates: Starchy (Carb-Starch)	1 Serving
Beans	1 cup
Rice	1 cup
Oatmeal	1 cup
Cereals (natural)	1 cup
Corn	1 cup or 1 ear
Pancakes	2 (5" diameter)
Waffles	2 (5" diameter)
Potato	1 medium size
Pasta	6 oz.
Rye bread	1 slice
100% whole-wheat bread	1 slice
Muffins (no-fat)	1
Crackers	4
Chips (low-fat)	8
Rice cakes	1

Carbohydrates: Fibrous (Carb-Fibrous)	1 Serving
Most vegetables, including:	
Alfalfa sprouts	1 cup
Beets	1 cup

Broccoli	1 cup
Cabbage	1 cup
Carrots	1, average size
Cauliflower	1 cup
Corn	1 cup, or 1 ear
Cucumber	1 cup
Leaf lettuce	1 cup
Mushrooms	1 cup
Onions	1 cup
Tomato	1 cup

CARBOHYDRATES: SIMPLE (CARB-SIMPLE)   1 SERVING

All fruit, including:	
Apple	1
Banana	1
Blueberries	1 cup
Cantaloupe	1/4
Cherries	1 cup
Dates	1/4 cup
Figs	1/4 cup
Grapefruit	1/2
Grapes (red, green, purple)	1/4 cup
Melon	2" slice
Orange	1 average size
Papaya	½
Peach	1 average size
Pear	1 average size
Pineapple	1" slice
Plum	2 average size
Raisins	¼ cup
Strawberries	1 cup
Ice Cream (no-fat)	¼ cup
Sherbet (low-sugar)	½ cup
Yogurt (no-fat, low-sugar)	6–8 oz.

BEVERAGES	1 SERVING
Water	At least 48–64 oz. daily
Fruit juice	8 oz.
Vegetable juice	8 oz.
Skim milk	8 oz.
Coffee/tea	8 oz.
Soft drinks (no sugar)	8 oz.

FATS	1 SERVING
Butter	1 tbsp
Nuts	¼ cup
Oils	2 tbsp
Seeds	½ cup
Sour cream	1 oz.
Peanut butter	2 tbsp
Mayonnaise	1 tbsp

MISCELLANY	1 SERVING
Spices and herbs	As desired
Mustard	As desired
Vinegar	As desired
BBQ sauce	2 tbsp
Teriyaki Sauce	2 tbsp
Soy sauce (low-sodium)	2 tbsp

Supplements	1 Serving
Colloidal minerals	1–2 oz. daily
Protein	20 grams 1–2 times daily
Pantocrine	1–3 capsules daily for 23 days, 7 days off
Phytonutrients	1–2 capsules 2–3 times daily
Antioxidants	1–2 capsules 2–3 times daily
Creatine	5 grams daily
Vitamin C	1,000 mg daily
Melatonin	1–3 mg before bed, occasional use
Enzymes	1–2 capsules with every meal
Chromium picolinate	200 mcg daily
L-carnitine	300 mgs daily
Omega-3, evening primrose oil	1 tbsp or 1 capsule daily

Exercise

The exercise component of each template outlines the frequency, duration and intensity of the physical activities that will help you reach your health and fitness goals. *Frequency* indicates how often you'll exercise each week. *Duration* refers to the length of each workout. *Intensity* is expressed as a resistance or a target heart rate.

While I have designed an integrated mix of aerobic and strength/anaerobic activities, you will choose the *specific* workout elements best suited to your schedule, your budget, and your exercise preferences. The following guidelines will help.

- Establish a convenient, realistic, and, above all, regular activities schedule. Any time of day or night is suitable for exercise, but, based on average metabolic activity ranges, late afternoon or early evening is best and often most practical (by a narrow, hardly significant margin).
- Be consistent in your exercise efforts. A workout every two or three weeks is not only useless, it may be dangerous. Sudden sustained exertion can severely damage an unprepared, poorly conditioned body.
- Start your exercise process with modest exertion and increase your workload gradually. I want to stress that you should approach all activities at your own pace. Don't ever feel obligated to perform at the level of others. You are restructuring *your* body, and you must allow time for that unique body to work through a conditioning period. You probably can't wait to get going full tilt, but there is an adaptation sequence that every body engineer must experience as the body adjusts itself to new patterns of activity. Once you've completed an adequate conditioning period, you can become more aggressive and seek tougher challenges.
- Accept the fact that on some days you simply won't be able to exercise as intensely as you'd like. No one's body is equally willing each day. Pay attention when your body

rebels, but come back fresh and determined for your next session.

- Never exercise while you are suffering from an infection. Most bacterial and viral infections are exacerbated by strenuous activity.
- Choose activities you enjoy, but avoid those that your body simply isn't ready for yet.
- Include as many different activities as possible in your exercise plan.
- Regardless of the activities you select for your exercise plan, on days when both anaerobics and aerobics are scheduled, complete your anaerobic activity first—to accelerate the "burn" and "afterburn" benefits of your exercise sessions.
- Enhance your aerobic activities with moderate-to-high-intensity "bursts." This Interval Aerobics approach will maximize the value of your aerobics.
- As you progress through your Body Engineering project, you're going to find yourself wanting to increase the intensity and duration of your workouts. Step up your activity levels gradually and defer to your body's most efficient communication device—pain. If something you're doing hurts, stop.
- Don't allow your body to become dehydrated during exercise. Drink plenty of water—the fluid your body absorbs best—before and after your activities. Whenever you exercise for more than forty-five minutes, drink water and carbo mixes during your workout as well.

Body engineering is a personal process, individually designed and self-directed—which is why I've listed an extensive buffet of activities that you can use to meet your unique fitness goals. The information that follows will provide you with a number of "workout" options you can mix and match to suit your schedule and lifestyle. This list is by no means all-inclusive. You can, and should, make your own list of all the things you like to do that are convenient, fun, and physical. It's easy to prevent boredom if you rotate several different activities throughout the course of the Body Engineering process. Spice up your exercise routine with as many choices as possible. There's no law that says exercise can't be fun.

As you review the survey of exercise options that you can use to fashion your personal workout plan, note that several of the aerobic activities easily become anaerobic with sufficient increases in intensity and that several of the anaerobic exercises have aerobic elements.

IMPORTANT! Even the most basic movements can be dangerous when muscles and joints are cold and stiff. To reduce the risk of muscle strain, ligament injuries, or joint damage, and to achieve maximum value from your workouts, begin each Body Engineering activity session with flexibility exercises. Warming up and stretching before strenuous physical activity allows you to dispel the tensions of the day and focus on your upcoming workout. A well-planned preparation routine also produces significant physiological benefits. Each degree you raise body heat increases the metabolic rate in muscle cells by 13 percent. A ten-to-fifteen-minute warm-up brings your body to an ideal work temperature. If you repeat your flexibility routine after your workout, the cool-down process that occurs will result in less soreness and stiffness after exercise ends. The flexibility test exercises you completed in chapter 4 are an excellent pre- and post-workout protocol. If you wish, you may perform your flexibility routine even on your "rest" days.

Creating an Active Lifestyle

With only some minor changes in your daily habits, you can incorporate useful calorie-burning movement into every aspect of your daily routine.

First, stop driving around searching for the perfect parking place. Weather permitting, always park your car in the farthest corner of the parking lot. And after grocery shopping, always return your cart to the least convenient collection island.

Develop an aversion for elevators. Whenever possible, use the stairs. Stair climbing can do wonders for the hips, buttocks, and legs. In fact, stair climbing would be an excellent addition to your activity selection list. If you feel energetic, take two steps at a time for an even more productive mini-workout.

Revise your approach to household chores and yard work. Try power lawn mowing, power vacuuming, or power garage cleaning. Make the most of these activities whenever you do them. When you can't find the time for formal exercise, invest a little more energy into your weekly chores. Chopping wood and moving furniture are excellent aerobic activities, and there's very little difference between the arm rotations you perform while dusting and the upper arm work you do in an aerobic class.

Daily activities can successfully be used to burn fat calories and enhance health. Don't choose the easy, lazy option for doing anything. Push yourself at every opportunity. You'll be pleasantly surprised at how quickly your body will accept your new habits. Walk the dog or play with the kids. Having children or an active pet can be like living with a personal trainer.

Aerobic Exercise Menu

Aerobic class	Jogging
Basketball	Rowing
Biking	Running
Climbing	Skating (ice or in-line)
Cross-country skiing	Swimming
Dance	Walking

Anaerobic Exercise Menu

MUSCLE GROUP	ACTIVITY
Chest	Bench Press
	Incline Flye
	Bench Dip
	Push-Up
	Flye
Shoulders	Upright Press
	Lateral Raise
	Upright Row
Biceps	Curl
	Alternating Curl
Triceps	Bench Dip
	Push-Back
	Single Arm Triceps Press
Legs/Quads	Squat
	Split Squat
	Lunge
	Leg Kick
Hips	Knee-Up
	Lunge
	Hip Roll
	Leg Kick
Buttocks	Back Leg Raise
	Back Leg Push
	Hip Roll

Inner thighs/Hamstrings	V-In
	Leg Curl
	Stiff Leg Dead Lift
Calves	Calf Raise
Upper back	Bent-Over Row
	Single Arm Row
	Shrug
Lower back	Hyperextension
	Single Back Leg Kick-n-Reach
	Stiff Leg Dead Lift
Upper abs	Crunch
	Crunch Pivot
Lower abs	V-Sit
	Reverse Crunch
Obliques	Oblique Twist
	Seated Side Bend
Total body	Pull Squat (Standing)
	Pull Squat (Seated)
	Flip Press

ANAEROBIC EXERCISE DESCRIPTIONS

Experiment with different weights until you find the resistance that enables you to fail within the range of repetitions listed in your template. For example, the weight is too light if you could easily do more than the suggested *maximum* number of repetitions per set. Conversely, the weight is too heavy if you can't complete the suggested *minimum* number of repetitions per set.

Chest

Bench Press

Lie faceup on a bench. Hold the dumbbells directly over your chest with arms locked. Slowly lower the weights simultaneously until your hands are at chest level. Push the weights back up to arm's length.

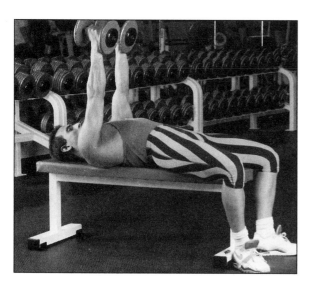 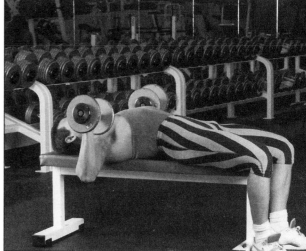

Incline Flye

Lie face-up on a bench set at a 45-degree angle. Grasp a dumbbell in each hand and hold with extended arms above your chest. Lower the dumbbells slowly, flaring them to the sides until they are at chest level. Squeeze the dumbbells back up until your arms are fully extended.

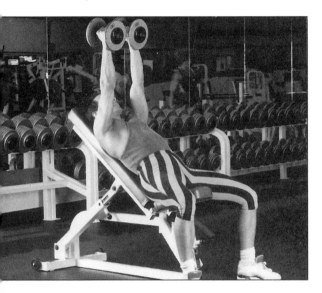 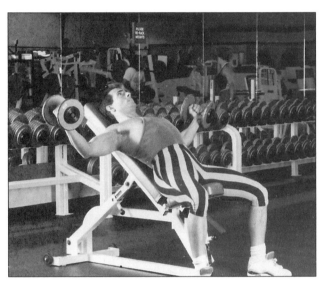

Push-Up

Lie facedown on a mat or the floor and place your hands underneath your shoulders, adjacent to your chest. While keeping your body rigid, push yourself up until your arms lock. Now lower yourself slowly until your chest slightly touches the floor.

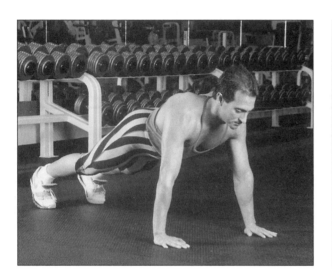 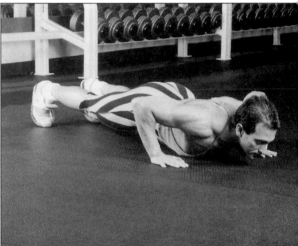

Flye

Lie faceup on a bench, feet flat against the floor. Grasp a dumbbell in each hand and hold with extended arms above your chest. Lower the dumbbells slowly, flaring them to the sides until they are at chest level. Squeeze the dumbbells back up until your arms are fully extended.

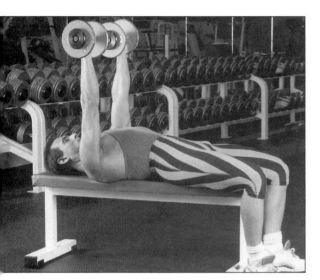 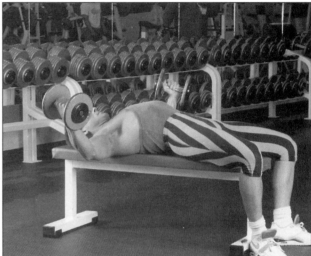

Shoulders

Upright Press

Sit upright at the edge of a bench or chair with a dumbbell in each hand at shoulder height. Push the weights straight upward until arms lock. Hold for a count of 1, then lower slowly to starting position.

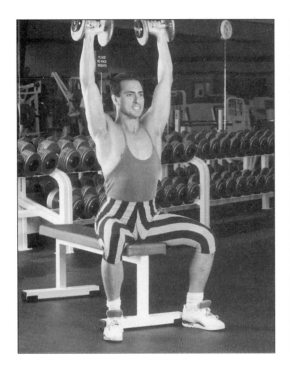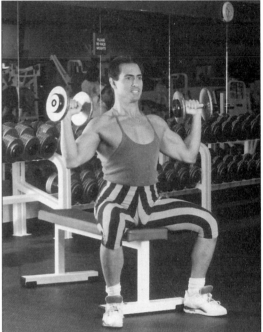

Lateral Raise

Stand upright with a dumbbell in each hand in front of your thighs, palms facing each other. Bend elbows slightly and lift the dumbbells to the level of the top of your head while turning your palms out. Hold for a count of 1 and slowly lower to starting position.

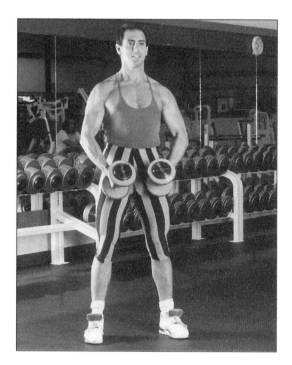 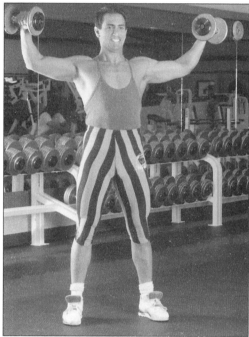

Upright Row

Stand upright with a dumbbell in each hand in front of your thighs, palms facing your thighs. Lift both elbows simultaneously until the dumbbells are raised to chin level. Hold for a count of 1, then lower to starting position.

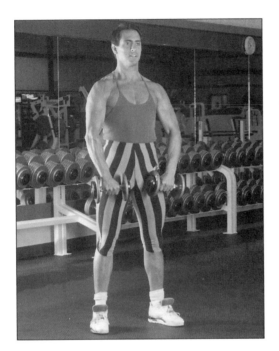 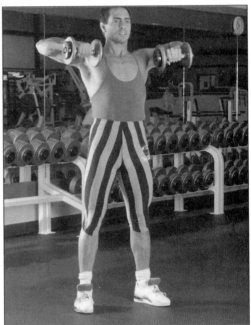

Triceps

Bench Dip

Sit on the side of a very sturdy, stable bench with your hands firmly placed beside your hips. Keeping your arms locked, extend your feet far enough to pull your buttocks off the bench. Lower yourself slowly until your arms are bent at 90 degrees. Pause for a count of 1, then push back up to arm-lock position.

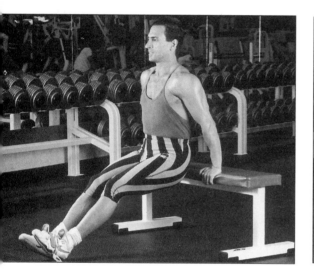 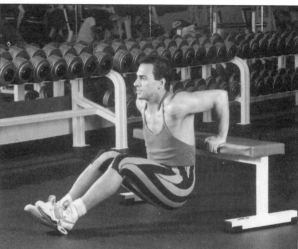

Push-Back

Place your left hand and knee on a bench so that your upper body is parallel to the bench. Hold a dumbbell in your right hand at chest height. Push the weight behind you as far as possible and hold for a count of 1. Slowly return to starting position. Switch sides and repeat.

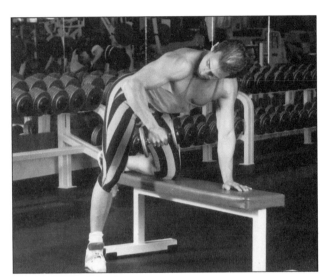 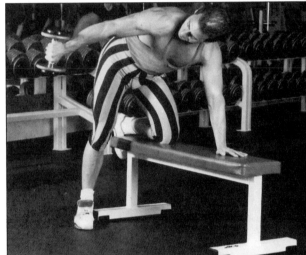

Single Arm Triceps Press

Lie faceup on a bench, feet flat against the floor. Grasp a dumbbell with your right hand and fully extend that arm above your chest. Support your right elbow with your left hand. Lower the weight to your right shoulder and return upward. Switch sides and repeat.

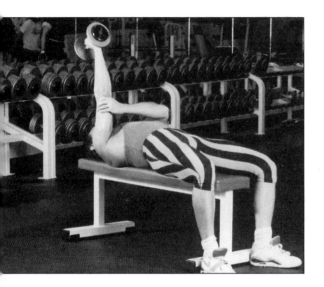 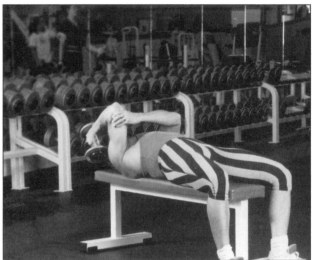

Biceps

Curl

Stand upright with a dumbbell in each hand with arms at your side, palms facing forward. Simultaneously curl the dumbbells toward your shoulders by flexing at the elbows. Hold for a count of 1, then slowly lower to starting position.

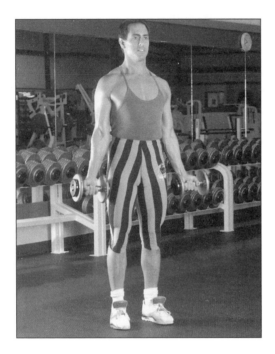 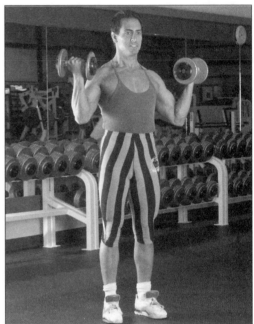

Alternating Curl

Same as for the Curl (above) but alternate between right and left arms.

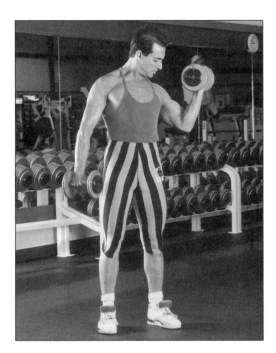 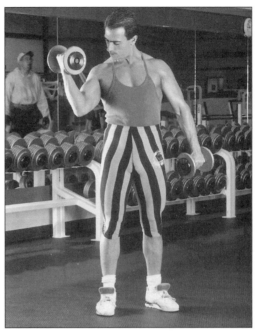

Squats

Stand upright with your feet a little more than shoulder width apart, toes slightly pointed outward. Keeping your back straight, bend at your hips and knees to lower yourself until your thighs are parallel to the floor. Raise your arms in front of you for balance. Hold for a count of 1 and push upward until your legs straighten.

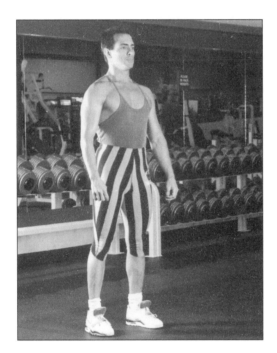 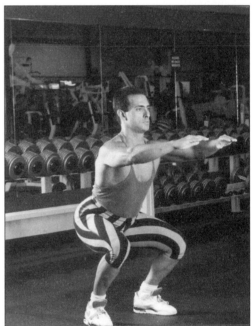

Split Squats

Stand upright with your feet a little more than shoulder width apart. Place your left foot about 2 feet forward of your right foot. Bend your left knee while dropping your right knee to the floor. Push up to split stance. Complete all the required reps before switching to the other side and repeat.

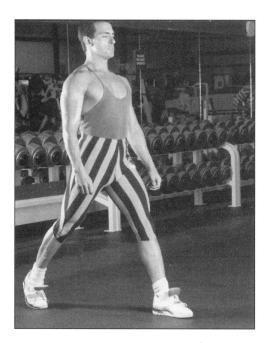
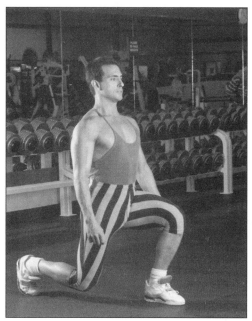

Lunges

Stand upright with your feet a little more than shoulder width apart. Extend your left foot forward about 2 feet. Bend your left knee while dropping your right knee to the floor. Push back with your left leg to return to starting position. Switch sides and repeat.

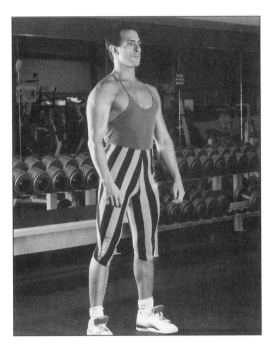 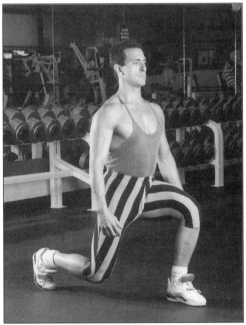

Leg Kicks

Sit on the edge of a chair or bench and grasp the sides for stability. Lean slightly backward, keeping your back straight and chest up. Kick (but do not snap) your right foot upward, then return to starting position while you kick your left foot.

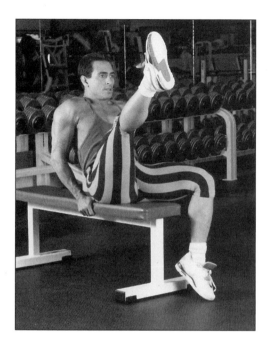 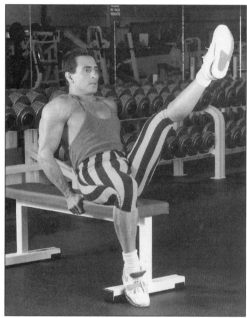

Hips

Knee-Up

Sit on the edge of a chair or bench and hold onto the sides. Lean slightly backward and slowly lift your right knee toward your chest. Lower slowly and repeat with the left leg.

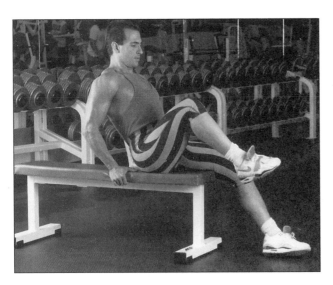 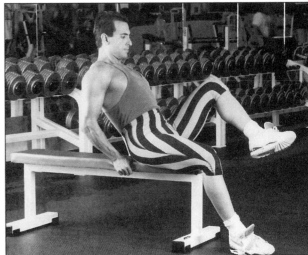

Hip Roll

Stand upright, hands on hips, at the end of a bench or any object at least 12 inches off the floor. Slowly lift the leg closest to the bench and swing it forward, then over and around the bench. Repeat in the opposite direction by lifting your leg to the rear and swinging it over and around to the front of the bench. Switch sides and repeat.

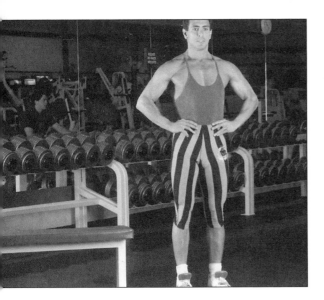 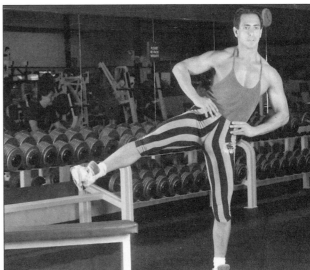

Back Leg Raise

Lie facedown on a bench so that your hips are just off the edge. Extend your legs as far apart as possible and straighten your knees. Grasping the front sides of the bench for stability, lift both legs upward, squeezing your heels together. Hold for a count of 1 and return to starting position.

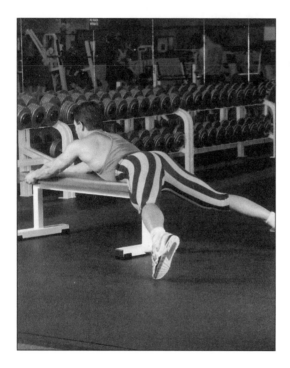 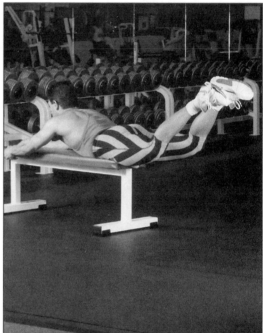

Back Leg Push

While kneeling on all fours on a mat or the floor, bring your left
knee toward your left elbow, then fully extend your leg behind you.
Hold for a count of 1 and repeat. Do not allow your foot to drag
on the floor. Switch legs and repeat.

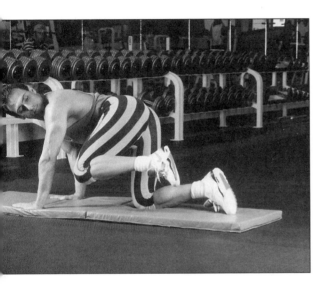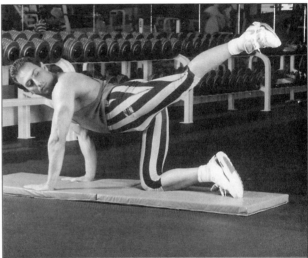

V-In

Lie faceup on a mat or the floor with legs spread and knees slightly bent. Place your hands palm-down under the small of your back. Slowly squeeze your legs inward and upward until your heels meet about 12 to 24 inches off the floor. Hold for a count of 1, then slowly lower to starting position.

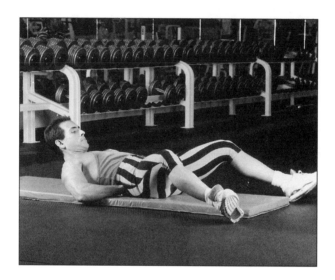

Leg Curl

Standing upright, lift your left foot off the floor and curl your heel as close as possible to your buttocks. Squeeze and hold the position for a count of 1. Straighten your leg slowly but don't let it touch the floor. Alternate between legs.

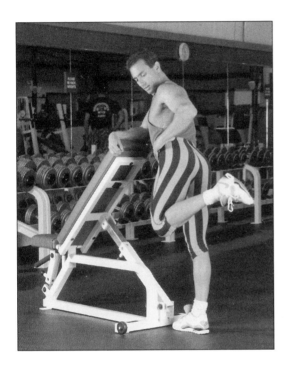

Bent-Over Row

Stand upright with a dumbbell in each hand at arm's length. Slowly bend forward at the waist and lock your back, keeping your knees slightly bent. Slowly pull the weights upward to the sides of your chest. Slowly lower the weights until your arms straighten.

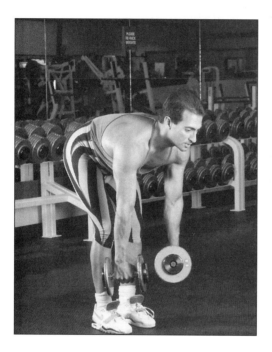 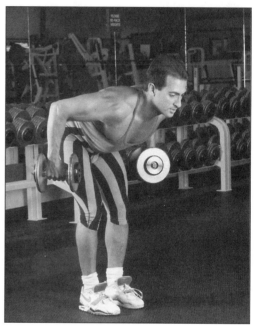

Single Arm Row

Stand beside a bench and place your left hand and knee on the bench with your right leg on the floor. Hold a dumbbell in your right hand with arm fully extended downward. Pull the weight upward to the side of your chest and hold for a count of 1. Slowly lower your arm to starting position. Switch sides and repeat.

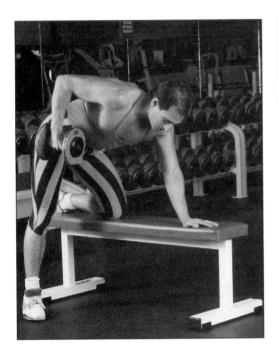 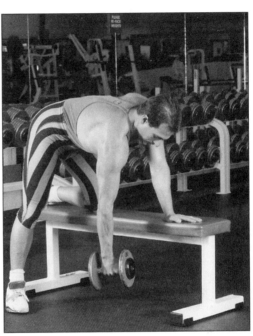

Shrug

Stand upright with a dumbbell in each hand in front of your thighs, palms facing your thighs. Keeping your elbows rigid, shrug your shoulders as high as possible. Hold for a count of 1, then repeat.

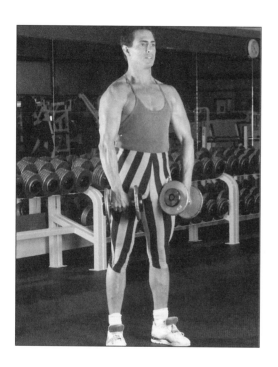 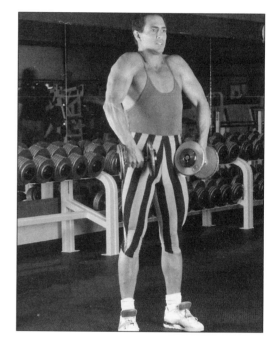

Lower Back

Hyperextension

Lie facedown on a mat or the floor with your hands clasped behind your lower back. Slowly lift your head and upper back just a few inches and hold for a count of 1. Lower yourself slowly to starting position.

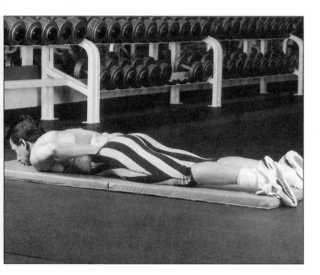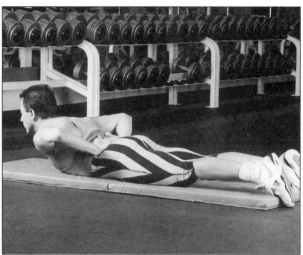

Single Back Leg Kick-n-Reach

Get on all fours on a mat or the floor. Lift and extend your right arm forward while extending your left leg back and up, parallel to the floor. Hold your arm and leg in the highest position possible for a count of 1, then slowly lower to starting position. Repeat with your left arm and right leg.

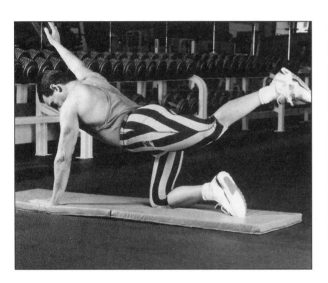 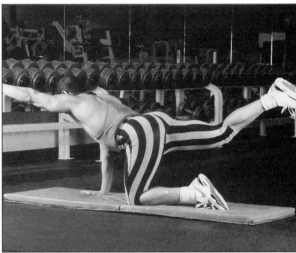

Stiff Leg Dead Lift

Stand upright, arms at your sides, with a dumbbell in each hand. Slowly bend forward at the waist, bending knees slightly. Lean as far as possible, preferably touching the weights to the floor. Slowly return to the starting position.

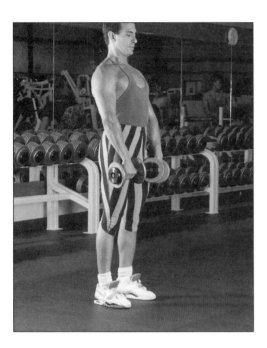 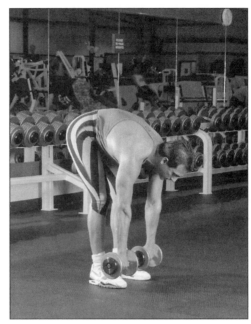

Crunch

Lie faceup on a mat or the floor with your hands resting on your upper abdominals. Bend your knees until your feet are flat against the floor. Lift your upper back 2 to 3 inches from the floor and hold for a count of 1. Lower yourself slowly to starting position.

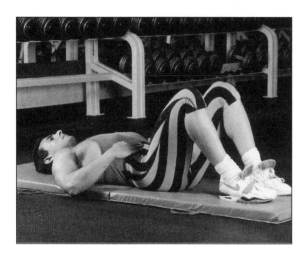
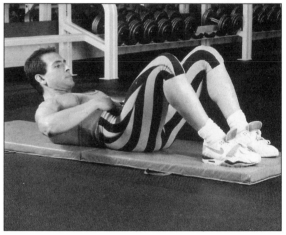

Crunch Pivot

Lie faceup on a mat or the floor. Bend your knees until your feet are flat against the floor, arms extended at your sides. Lift your upper back about 2 to 3 inches from the floor and hold while twisting your torso to the left and right.

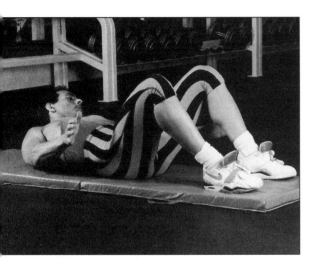 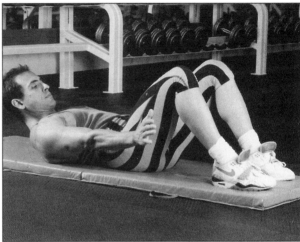

V-Sit

Sit at the edge of a chair or bench and hold onto the sides. Lean slightly backward and slowly pull both knees to your chest. Hold for a count of 1, then slowly lower to starting position.

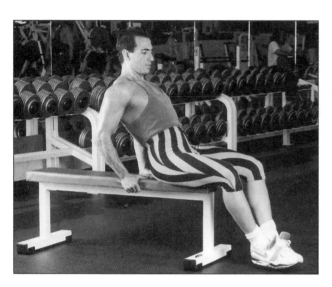 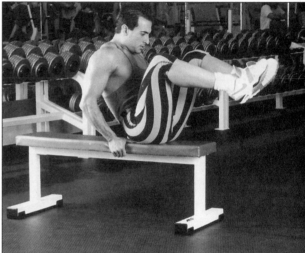

Reverse Crunch

Lie faceup on a mat or the floor with your hands resting on your lower abdominals. Pull your knees to your chest, trying to lift your buttocks off the floor, and hold for a count of 1. Return to starting position.

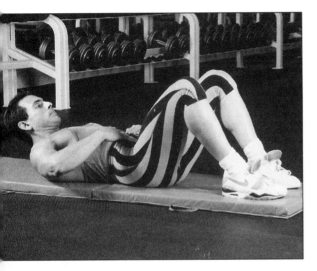 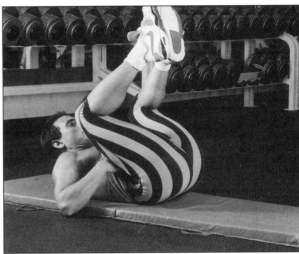

Obliques

Oblique Twist

Sit upright on a mat or the floor, knees bent, heels together. Rotate your torso from right to left while pumping your arms.

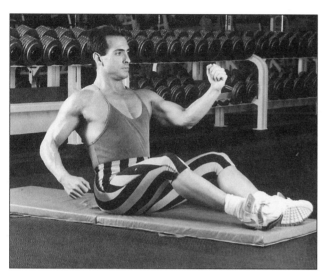
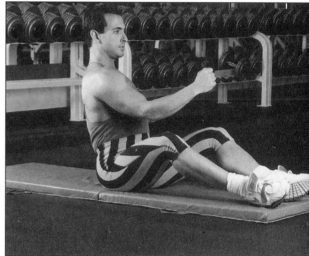

Seated Side Bend

Sit upright on a mat or the floor with your legs spread as wide as possible. Your arms should be shoulder height and bent at a 90-degree angle. Bend a few inches from one side to the other in pendulum-like fashion.

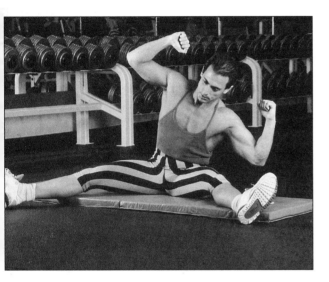 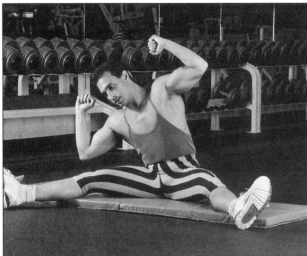

Calf Raise

Stand upright with the balls of both feet on an elevated object like a small box, book, or step. It might be helpful to hold onto a fixed object for support. Lower your heels until you feel a good stretch, then push up on your toes and raise your heels as high as possible. Hold for a count of 3 and repeat.

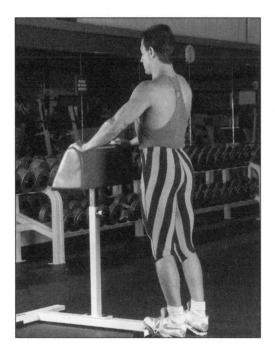
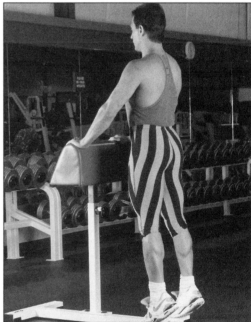

Total Body

Pull Squat (Standing)

Stand upright with feet at shoulder width. Place a dumbbell along the outside of each foot. From the upright position, bend at the waist and knees to reach down and grasp each weight. Lift the weights overhead to full arm extension, hold for a count of 1, and slowly lower to starting position.

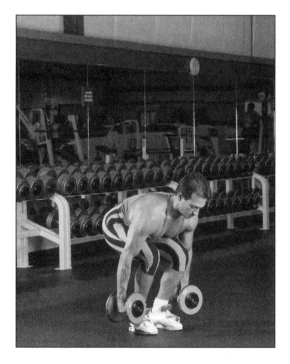
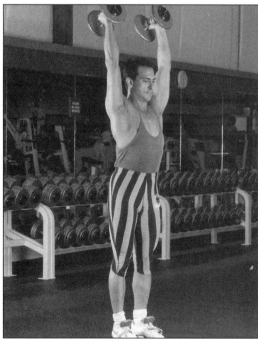

Pull Squat (Seated)

Sit on the edge of a bench or chair. Place a dumbbell along the outside of each foot. From the upright position, bend at the waist to reach down and grasp each weight. Lift the weights overhead to full arm extension, hold for a count of 1, and slowly lower to starting position.

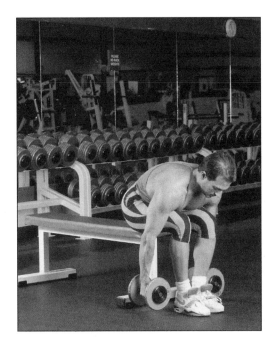 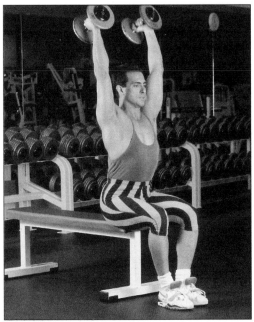

Flip Press

Stand upright, arms at your sides, with a dumbbell in each hand. Lift your right hand toward your right shoulder, then press it overhead until your arm straightens. While slowly lowering your right hand to its starting position, repeat the procedure with your left hand.

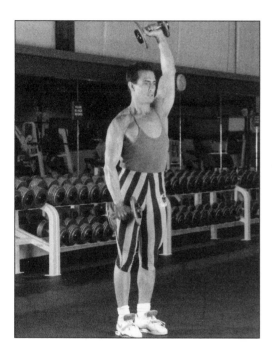 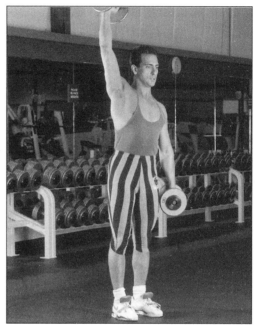

MILLIE AND MARTY

For an illustration of how the Body Engineering templates can assist in the planning and implementation of your physical renovation process, here is a comparison of Millie and Marty, two fitness novices with quite different needs and objectives.

Millie, a thirty-something elementary school teacher, knows she is too heavy. She has been gaining weight steadily since the birth of her son three years ago. Millie's self-assessment tests confirmed that her body fat percentage is approaching a level she finds embarrassing, and her aerobic capacity is well below the level she needs to keep pace with her three-year-old and the responsibilities of her career.

Millie chooses the Weight Loss template. As she reviews her nutrition choices, she realizes that she can meet her nutritional goals without drastic changes in her eating habits. Millie's customized nutrition template looks like this:

MILLIE'S NUTRITION TEMPLATE

	OPTION 1	OPTION 2
MEAL 1	1 banana 1 cup fat-free yogurt 2 eggs	1 cup oatmeal 1 grapefruit Coffee
SNACK	¼ cup figs 1 orange Tea	Lettuce and tomato salad Fat-free dressing 8 oz. orange juice
MEAL 2	4 oz. cottage cheese Cucumber and onion salad Vinegar and oil dressing 8 oz. vegetable juice	8 oz. turkey ¼ cup grapes 1 cup corn 8 oz. orange juice
MEAL 3	1 slice whole-wheat bread 1 tbsp butter Mushrooms and broccoli 8 oz. chicken 8 oz. diet soda	8 oz. fish Coleslaw (1 cup cabbage, 1 shredded carrot, mayonnaise, mustard, salt and pepper) 8 oz. diet soda

SNACK	Salad
	Fat-free/sugar-free dressing
	Iced tea
		1 potato stuffed with
		    mushrooms and
		    cauliflower
		Fat-free sour cream
		Iced tea

Winter is approaching the midwestern state where Millie lives, so she determines that her initial aerobic sessions will be spent pedaling a stationary bike. She finds a barely used model at a garage sale and buys it for forty dollars. Because Millie is following the Weight Loss template, her strength program looks like this:

Millie's Strength Template

WORKOUT 1		WORKOUT 2	
Total body	Standing Pull Squat	Total body	Flip Press
Chest	Push-Up	Legs	Squat
Legs	Leg Kick	Upper abs	Crunch
Shoulders	Lateral Raise	Lower abs	V-Sit
Hips	Hip Roll	Buttocks	Back Leg Push
Biceps	Curl	Triceps	Push-Back
Upper abs	Crunch Pivot	Inner thighs	V-In
Upper back	Shrug	Shoulders	Upright Row
Hamstrings	Leg Curl	Calves	Calf Raise
Obliques	Seated Side Bend	Lower back	Hyperextension

After five weeks of Body Engineering, Millie conducts her own process review. She concludes that her nutrition plan is working well but admits that she is becoming bored with her stationary bike. She also believes that she has become strong enough to accept the challenge of free weights and resistance exercise machinery.

When she realizes that it's time to revise her activity template, Millie purchases a trial membership at a local health club operated by the county's parks and recreation department. The club's fitness center houses treadmills, steppers, rowing and cross-country skiing machines, and a wide array of free weights and other strength equipment as well as a swimming pool and an indoor track.

By the time her temporary status expires, Millie has tried everything the health club has to offer. She likes the variety of activities available and decides to become a member. Access to the fitness center's resources permits Millie to consider several different strength/anaerobic circuits, and almost unlimited aerobic exercise options.

As Millie's Body Engineering process moves forward, she gravitates toward activities she likes, and eliminates those she finds awkward or uncomfortable or dull. She makes the appropriate alterations in her activity template.

If Millie stays with her renovation plan and continues her progress, she will make frequent changes in the intensity and duration levels of her activity template. She may also change her exercise choices to keep her workouts fresh and challenging.

Marty, a soft, undersized auto mechanic, is not the least bit interested in downsizing. He realizes that he is already too scrawny and too weak to cope with the physical demands of his daily life. Tired of always being tired, and fed up with the string of stupid nicknames he has acquired at the engine shop where he works, Marty is determined to add muscle mass and strength.

Marty chooses the Weight Gain template. His nutrition plan calls for four meals and one or two snacks each day. Because the body builds muscle from proteins and carbohydrates, Marty needs a steady flow of these foods throughout the day. No one Marty's size can consume the calories he'll need during the initial stages of his renovation process, so he adds a number of supplements to his eating plan. His nutrition template looks like this:

MARTY'S NUTRITION TEMPLATE

	OPTION 1	OPTION 2
MEAL 1	8 oz. cottage cheese 2 sliced peaches 3 slices whole-wheat toast 1 tbsp butter Coffee	4-egg omelet with mushrooms and green peppers 1 slice rye toast 1 tbsp butter 1 cup cold cereal 1 cup skim milk
SNACK	1 orange 1 apple 8 oz. vegetable juice	Salad Vinegar and oil dressing 4 oz. diced low-fat cheese

MEAL 2	2 chicken breasts
	1 potato
	1 tbsp. sour cream
	1 muffin
	1 diet soda
	Protein shake
		Hero sandwich
		(1 French roll,
		4 oz. turkey,
		4 oz. ham,
		2 oz. cheese,
		onions, green peppers and
		  mushrooms, mayonnaise
		  and mustard)
		Iced tea
		Protein shake

MEAL 3	8-oz. cheeseburger 1 bun 1 ear sweet corn ½ cup fat-free ice cream Iced tea	8 oz. cottage cheese 2 cups strawberries 8 crackers 1 diet soda

MEAL 4	8 jumbo shrimp Cocktail sauce 2 cups rice Salad 8 oz. apple juice	1 New York strip 6 oz. pasta 1 dinner roll Salad 8 oz. apple juice
SNACK	Cheese and crackers Water	Chef's salad with 8 oz. sliced turkey, 2 oz. cubed cheese, and lettuce Crackers Milk

Aware that weight training offers the most effective route to functional weight gain, Marty converts a basement storage area to a home gym and purchases a set of weights.

Marty's Weight Gain template recommends three weekly workouts focused on weight training. Because Marty needs increased muscle size as well as strength, he initially programs six to twelve repetitions of each exercise, with workloads that impose moderate to heavy resistance. The aerobic portion of Marty's template calls for sessions of fifteen to twenty minutes. His strength template looks like this.

Marty's Strength Template

Workout 1		Workout 2		Workout 3	
Chest	Bench Press	Total Body	Pull Squat (Seated)	Total body	Flip Press
Chest	Incline Flye	Legs	Squat	Shoulders	Upright Press
Chest	Flye	Legs	Lunge	Shoulders	Upright Row
Upper back	Bent-Over Row	Hamstrings	Leg Curl	Shoulders	Lateral Raise
Upper back	Shrug	Calves	Calf Raise	Triceps	Bench Dip
Biceps	Curl	Lower back	Hyperextension	Triceps	Push-Back
Biceps	Alternating Curl	Upper abs	Crunch		
		Lower abs	V-Sit		
		Obliques	Oblique Twist		

Within two weeks after he begins his reconstruction project, Marty notices dramatic improvement in his strength and energy levels. Shortly thereafter, the structural change he has implemented becomes apparent to the guys down at the garage.

Engineering is a practical, empirical process—a series of adjustments, a sequence of trial and error, and trial and success. Your body is a living, dynamic organism, and so is your renewal process. Expect change. In fact, welcome it. The Body Engineering templates you have at your disposal are free-form structures. Review your nutrition and exercise plans frequently, check your progress against your baseline data, and revise your templates whenever the need—or the desire—arises.

CHAPTER SIX

Vision and Reality

Using Your Mind to Change Your Body

Every engineering effort ever undertaken—from the most trivial to the most complex—began with a vision. Not a fantasy, or a technical diagram, or a stylized artist's rendering, the gifted engineer's vision is a crystal-clear, multidimensional mental image.

In a similar fashion, the skilled body engineer experiences his or her new body, and new life, long before either exists . . .

A sleek trim shadow gliding effortlessly along a golden tropical beach.

A sinewy hiker exploring the north rim of the Grand Canyon.

A powerful dad rowing his family across a deep blue Wisconsin lake.

A lean agile mom playing volleyball with her teenage daughters and their friends.

These are visions, not pipe dreams or delusions. These are glimpses of potential, images of a viable future.

The first chapters of this book surveyed the raw materials, knowledge, techniques, and planning skills you need to make your Body Engineering vision a flesh-and-blood reality. You know most of what you need to know to achieve your goals. While there are dozens of minor details you may need to work out before you can begin your renovation process, there's really only one major obstacle to overcome—a single but potentially formidable threat to success:

You.

The intricate and unique blend of attitude, outlook, fears, yearnings, needs, and beliefs that defines who you are must be reshaped and rechanneled to accommodate your Body Engineering goals. You are planning to change, to improve. The change you have in mind may be a minor lifestyle adjustment or a dramatic alteration of several perceptual and cognitive functions. It doesn't really matter. No change is possible until you choose to change, and no change will occur until you act to implement the decision to change.

Designing an effective Body Engineering process is not difficult. Depending on the current state of your relationship with yourself, generating the motivation necessary to build the body you've designed may pose more of a challenge.

To be effective, motivation must come from within. Depending on others—or external factors—as an impetus for change almost always results in failure.

The Body Engineering process is a vehicle for change. While its analytical components offer information you should be able to use to motivate yourself on an intellectual level, you must manage the psychological and emotional aspects of the changes you will be implementing. As I've stressed again and again, this is your process. You will be making all project decisions and controlling all project activities. You must supply the determination, time, and energy required to transform yourself from who you are now into who you want to be. You must align your priorities and create an engineering philosophy that has meaning and purpose. You must take charge.

Self-Motivation

Typically, the elements you will need to develop the self-motivation necessary for a successful body renovation effort include the following.

- *Desire.* Motivation begins with a sincere desire to achieve a goal. The body engineer's goal is to create a strong, healthy, aesthetically appealing, and efficient body.

- *Faith.* You must be convinced that it's possible to achieve your goals through the Body Engineering process. To assist you in establishing the degree of confidence you'll need for success, I guarantee that if you incorporate Body Engineering's basic principles into your life, you will experience meaningful improvement in your body's appearance and performance.

- *Hope.* No one can be motivated to pursue any course of action he or she believes to be futile. The fact that the Body Engineering process offers a practical, viable vehicle for reaching your goals should persuade you that you can reasonably expect a successful renovation and that your current physical condition is neither permanent nor unchangeable.

- *Responsibility.* Recognize that you and you alone are responsible for the success of your Body Engineering process. Welcome the challenge, see the process not as a burden, but as a valuable opportunity. Trust yourself with the responsibility for your life and realize that you have within you all the resources you need to reach your goals.

- *Action.* Continuous positive action is essential to maintain the energy, self-confidence, and motivation necessary to move the Body Engineering process forward. Begin slowly, one small step at a time. Proceed at your own pace, but, by all means, proceed.

Embracing Change

Change is inevitable. Every element of our world is constantly reshaping and redefining itself—from the smallest subatomic particles to the universe itself. Your body's cellular structure has completely remodeled itself in the past twelve months.

Recall how you looked, felt, thought, and acted five or ten years ago. You're not the same person you were in high school or on your wedding day or the day your first child was born. You've changed. We all have. Life is a series of never-ending changes.

Although change is an inherent, completely natural aspect of existence, many humans hate and fear it. Even when we're dissatisfied or unhappy with our current condition, we avoid or resist making the renovations and improvements we know we need to make.

A serious commitment to the Body Engineering process will require changes in certain habits and lifestyle choices that you believe you enjoy. It's difficult to change comfortable or pleasant routines, even when we know we must, and admit we must, and know why we must. Change makes us apprehensive because change always introduces elements of the unknown into our lives. Unknowns tend to make us emotionally anxious, regardless of the assurances and guarantees we receive, and despite our intellectual acceptance of the need to change.

Ironically, when your health and fitness are at issue, refusal or postponement of change for the better pretty much assures that you'll change for the worse. Your body will continue its lifelong cycle of change. Resisting these changes is like trying to wrestle a river. The real question becomes not how to avoid change, but how best to direct the transformation.

By completing the self-assessment tests, you took the first step to meaningful change—*you have accurately identified the physical improvements you would like to make.*

The Body Engineering process (or any improvement, construction, or renovation effort) requires time, attention, expense, inconvenience, and, frankly, some degree of inner strength. A sign that you're ready for the challenges of the change process is that you stop searching for something or someone to change your life, and begin looking within yourself. *Emotional readiness for change is wanting to change, not simply the feeling that you should change.*

Body Engineering offers you the freedom to act on your own behalf. Self-initiated changes are made on your own terms, at your own pace. The total control the body engineer exerts throughout the process promotes effort, desire, satisfaction, and self-confidence. As you become aware that you are indeed in charge, the natural apprehension that change usually induces is dissipated. As you decide how you'll implement your project plan, you ll discover a wide array of exercise and nutrition options. The knowledge that these extensive choices are limited only by your own creativity and imagination should generate a feeling of freedom and allow you to relax. *Once you recognize that your improvement process is completely self-directed, the fear of change disappears.* A struggle *against* forsaking old familiar patterns becomes a campaign for rejuvenation.

Procrastination

When Beth launched her Body Engineering project, she was already action-oriented. Within days she absorbed the technical knowledge she needed, created a sensible eating plan, and melded a vigorous activities routine into her weekly schedule. When her process veered off track, she quickly made adjustments and moved forward. Within fourteen weeks Beth achieved her Body Engineering goals.

The renovation effort unfolded smoothly and successfully primarily because Beth had a great deal of experience with the dynamics of change. Beth is an ex-smoker and a recovering alcoholic. Along the way to becoming alcohol and nicotine free, Beth learned some hard and valuable lessons—among them the ability to overcome the human tendency to procrastinate. Long before adopting the Body Engineering approach, Beth had learned that action is necessary to solve problems and effect change.

Procrastination is a common trait. Almost everyone puts off doing what needs to be done at some point in his or her life. Often, we label chronic procrastinators as "lazy" or "lacking in discipline," or we decide that they simply can't manage their time very well.

We're wrong. Psychologists long ago discovered that procrastination is most often caused by suppressed fears or inspired by some type of emotional reward or secondary gain. Generally, the procrastinator either is not aware of his or her motives or chooses to ignore this awareness.

Ted was divorced and a hundred pounds overweight. He joined a weight-loss group, faithfully attended meetings, studied, took notes, and asked questions. The information Ted gathered became part of a wide-ranging, extremely intricate diet and exercise plan—a multicolored notebook bulging with charts and calendars and menus and schedules. But Ted's impressive plan was never converted into action.

Ted gradually realized that he was procrastinating. He became frustrated when he couldn't understand why he kept putting off what he thought he sincerely wanted to do.

Individual sessions with a psychologist revealed to Ted that fear was the source of his procrastination. He told the counselor that he was having trouble making friends and attributed this problem to his size. Without the extra pounds to blame, any rejection that came his way would be directed squarely at Ted the person. And that, Ted eventually admitted, would be devastating. Rather than expose himself to possible pain, Ted chose to procrastinate.

When Ted identified and understood his fear of rejection and of not having value as a person, he was only halfway home. Although his newfound awareness reduced his frustration, to address his weight problem effectively he still had to conquer his fears.

Typically, procrastination is an avoidance mechanism used to avoid such fears as these:

- *Success.* You consciously or unconsciously believe you won't be able to live with your new body. Your friends will expect more of you. Or they'll reject you or be angry with you for being "better" than they are.

- *Guilt.* You are convinced (at some emotional level) that you're not really worthy of the benefits your physical improvement will bring.
- *Self-esteem.* Once your self-improvement project is completed, you'll discover that you're not as good as everyone said you could be before the improvement occurred.
- *New challenges.* If you become fit and active, you'll be expected to try activities you can avoid now, and you'll fail in these new challenges.
- *The unknown.* If you change yourself, who knows what might happen? And who knows if you can live with the new you?

Some rewards that procrastinators usually seek include these:

- *Revenge.* Delaying action is seen as a passive-aggressive means for striking back at others who have made you angry or caused you pain.
- *Rebellion.* Taking your own sweet time to change is used as a mechanism for showing so-and-so (insert name of your favorite villain here) that he/she can't control you or force you to improve yourself.
- *Power.* Procrastination is used as a means of controlling others.
- *A miracle.* If you delay working on your problems long enough, someone or something will appear to save you the inconvenience, uncertainty, and effort of change.

While determining the cause of procrastination is probably helpful for long-term change, merely identifying the source of the problem isn't, by itself, very helpful. To overcome fears of success, failure, uncertainty, and so forth, you need a support system in which you feel comfortable enough to confront these apprehensions. If you are able to acknowledge the underlying causes of procrastination yourself, reassess your personal values and define new flexible directions for development. To alleviate self-imposed pressures and general uncertainty, lower your expectations of perfection to more realistic levels. Motivate yourself to continuous positive action by appreciating the small successes you'll encounter at each stage of the Body Engineering process.

In the early stages of your project, set goals that are reasonable for your current condition, and attainable in a short period of time. If, for instance, your ultimate goal is to lose fifty pounds, begin with a short-term goal of a five-to-ten-pound weight loss within the first month of your process. When you reach your first intermediate goal, you'll be able to see the light at the end of the tunnel.

According to behavioral psychologists, the emotional or subconscious influences that hamper our efforts to change are patterns that we have established ourselves based on internal cues (fears, rewards). Behaviorists believe that it's unnecessary to resort to intense psychoanalysis to improve an unsatisfactory condition or situation. All we need to do, they insist, is simply change our stimulation patterns until we recondition ourselves.

Behavioral techniques can be effective in the Body Engineering process as long as you remember that you (not the conditioning technique) are the source of improvement.

If you'd like to include a behavior modification component in your renovation process, you might start by keeping an hour-by-hour account of your eating and exercise patterns over a two-week period. Most people believe they are already aware of their behavior and thus won't benefit from keeping this record. Those who keep an accurate detailed log, however, are usually surprised at what they learn about themselves.

You may discover, for example, that you spend two hours a night watching television—usually with a plate of snacks within easy reach. To change that behavior pattern, you may decide to make a rule for yourself that food will only be eaten in the kitchen and that if you do anything while watching TV, it must be some type of exercise. If you examine all your behaviors, you may find several other opportunities for change.

Use a system of rewards to reinforce your new behavior patterns. Rewards can be anything you value (except large quantities of the wrong foods). For many of you, the improvements you'll note by comparing your baseline data to your current condition will be sufficient reward for your behavioral changes.

Assembling a Body Engineering Team

Because you spend so much of your time at home or at work, family members, friends, and colleagues can have considerable impact on your behavior, attitudes, and emotions. Strangely enough, the people in your life who care about you most are also the people most likely to sabotage your Body Engineering efforts. Although those close to you express a sincere willingness to help, their feelings about you, their misconceptions about what you really want, or their own needs and desires blind them to the negative effects they can exert on your renovation process. If their own body images or value systems are distorted, it becomes still harder for them to see you and your goals clearly.

Some people who share your life may find your self-improvement efforts threatening. The changes you desire may be seen as a catalyst for disruption in their lives or their relationships with you. As long as you stay as you are, these people feel secure. The changes you seek, on the other hand, could produce unknown consequences, and the unknown sparks anxiety.

Others close to you may welcome the changes you have in mind—and feel that they are long overdue. These people may become overzealous in their eagerness to help, stifling your efforts with overwhelming pressure and unrealistic expectations.

Cara, although she worked in a lawyer's office for most of her married life, found the time and energy to become her family's chief cook, housekeeper, and laundress. When Cara began a body renovation project that included classes, regular exercise, support group meetings, and an eating plan based on fresh healthful foods, her husband and two teenage daughters became noticeably upset. They didn't mind if Cara reengineered her body, but they didn't want her to stop waiting on them or changing *their* eating patterns. That would mean that Cara's family would have to do much more for themselves, and they wouldn't be eating their favorite meals unless they purchased and prepared their food themselves. Her family's reactions to Cara's self-improvement attempts were, predictably, nonsupportive and uncompromising. Cara felt overwhelmed, and she soon returned to her old self, feeling hopeless and bitter, unlikely to try again.

Bill's wife was overjoyed when he began his Body Engineering process. "You're too young to be soft and fat," she told him. Ten days into the project, Bill's wife had taken over. She constructed charts, designed and prepared meals, brought home fitness videos, and woke Bill up each morning at dawn for a four mile jog.

Bill soon found himself seething with resentment.

As Cara and Bill learned, your renovation efforts can be extremely vulnerable to the influence of others. Neither Cara nor Bill possessed the resolve and self-confidence needed to escape these obstacles.

To protect (and perhaps strengthen) your improvement process, take charge immediately. Prepare your family members and friends in an organized, consistent manner. Tell them what you are doing and why. When others know what to expect from you, they feel less threatened, even if they aren't especially happy about your plans for change.

One way to estimate the level of cooperation and support you may expect from those close to you is to approach family and friends as though you were assembling a Body Engineering team.

Start by paying attention to all the people with whom you interact regularly. Note how each approaches health and fitness. Evaluate their attitudes and values, and how they compare to yours. Realize that your relationship with some of these people may be part of the complex subconscious matrix that contributes to your current physical condition.

Explain your goals and plans to those likely to be affected by your Body Engineering process and let them know how they can aid, or at least not impede, your efforts. Going public with your intentions provides an interesting incentive for you and often supplies a valuable source of encouragement and discipline.

Your family and friends can be supportive and interested spectators, or helpful participants in your process. Regardless of their roles, remember that you are in charge. Accept useful suggestions but keep all decision-making powers for yourself. If a friend or family member becomes seriously interested in Body Engineering, by all means share what you've learned about the process. As an ancient axiom reminds us, we learn best when we teach.

Exercise and sensible eating are habits that are much easier to establish and maintain when a partner or a team shares your vision and commitment. Welcome allies in your renovation efforts but don't allow harmful competition to warp the process. Keep your goals in proper perspective. As we rebuild our bodies in a group setting of any kind, most of us experience a natural tendency to compare ourselves with others in the group. These kinds of comparisons can be helpful in setting realistic standards or as a motivational technique. Viewing Body Engineering as some sort of blood sport, however, can be destructive. If you see yourself "falling behind" a partner or team member, you may become depressed or frustrated and eventually find yourself not only alienated from your partner but fed up with the renovation process as well.

Be competitive only with yourself. Set your own pace and work toward your own goals. Use eating and exercise routines you find to be effective and realistic. Be appreciative, not envious, of whatever success your partners enjoy. And if you can't duplicate their results immediately, concentrate on matching their efforts. You will be rewarded.

Dealing with Setbacks

Every well-designed engineering process includes a series of fallback, recovery, and contingency plans. Veteran engineers expect glitches, delays, and problems. So should you.

Look into the future and imagine this scenario: You are following a sensible eating and exercise plan and beginning to feel good about yourself. Then one day, for no apparent reason, you lose focus. You become distracted by some special event or traumatic occurrence, or you simply decide to put your project aside for a couple of days or a week.

When you realize what has happened, you feel guilty or become depressed. Maybe, you suggest to yourself, you'll never develop the resolve needed to reach your renovation goals. Maybe you should give up.

Before you completely throw in the towel, remember that you wouldn't stop brushing your teeth if you missed a day. Don't overreact to missteps, errors, or setbacks. Forgive yourself and resume your improvement efforts immediately. Keep your mind on what lies ahead, not on what you're trying to leave behind. The fact is, no one, not even world-champion athletes, performs at the top of his or her form all the time. Michael Jordan, arguably the best basketball player ever, misses half the shots he attempts. The best hitters in baseball fail at the plate about two-thirds of the time.

Physical capability, energy levels, and mental attitude fluctuate dramatically over the course of any training effort. Far too many of us want to push continuously forward. Relax—that's not a practical goal. Expect frustrating periods during which your process seems stalled. In any nutritional or exercise process you will experience plateaus. It's the way your body adjusts to its new level of activity. Just when you think you won't improve, you'll find yourself making new gains. My favorite axiom may help you put things in perspective: *You can't see the grass growing, yet it is growing nonetheless.*

Be patient. Your body is changing, and in time these internal changes will begin to manifest themselves in your body's appearance and performance. Keep going, step by step. You can't expect to reverse years of neglect or indifference in a few weeks. You can't lose forty pounds without losing eight first, and you can't run three miles until you can run one.

Excuses, Excuses

Gauges mounted in the dashboard of your car alert you when you are running low on fuel, oil, or electrical energy. The list of excuses that follows serves a similar purpose and should be viewed as a clear indicator that your attitude about and commitment to your Body Engineering process may be in need of a tune-up. If you discover statements like these filling your mind or coming out of your mouth, recognize them for procrastination and try to come up with sensible counterarguments to keep yourself on track.

It's raining.
I'm depressed today.
We had company last night.
I'm tired.
I've just been too busy lately.
I feel kind of blah.
It's too cold.
It's too hot.
I'm bored.
My partner couldn't make it today.
I'm sore.
It's too late.
It's too early.
I need to be with a group.
I have no place to exercise.
It's the holidays.
I have a headache.
A day or two or three off isn't going to hurt anything.
It was dark when I got up this morning.
Nobody will exercise with me.
I forgot.
My kids needed me.
I read an article claiming exercise isn't good for everyone.
Sally never exercises and she's in great shape.

My doctor said if I run too much my uterus will fall.

It costs too much.

It was a special occasion.

I paid for that prime rib. I had to eat it.

My kids are impossible if we don't have sweets in the house.

The car turned in at McDonald's like there was a force field drawing it in.

I worked out hard today. I deserve a major treat.

Triple Fudge Ripple is the only thing that calms me down.

I didn't know it had forty-six grams of fat. I forgot to read the label.

I wasn't really paying attention to what I was eating.

I was angry and just didn't give a damn anymore.

It was junk food or nothing. I had no choice.

I'll work out twice tomorrow.

Try not to let excuses sideline you permanently. Every day is an opportunity to get going again. If too many excuses pile up, it may be time to look at your program closely—you may be setting too-high goals for yourself. Only you can determine what's right for yourself.

If you manage your Body Engineering process effectively, you'll move forward slowly at the beginning. As you progress, momentum will build. Each element of the process will affect the others. If you proceed steadily, adjusting the process as you go, you are likely to succeed at most of what you attempt. Remember not to denigrate yourself when you encounter difficulties. Allow yourself not to be perfect. Unrealistic expectations will strain your body and psyche and lead to burnout. Aim for a relaxed, balanced approach.

When you incorporate the advice or participation of others into your process, be careful that the aims of others don't supersede the goals you've set for yourself.

As the old song suggests, accentuate the positive. Don't fight yourself or the improvement process. Focus on what you are striving for, not on what you're giving up. Why worry about a sack of corn dogs and a couple of hours of TV sitcoms when years of active, vibrant life are awaiting you? If you immerse yourself in the renovation process rather than force yourself through it, your passage will be much smoother and more successful.

At times, your improvement process will seem to be exactly what it is—work. Accept the fact that you must earn the invaluable compensations that improved health and fitness will bring.

The fact that you are willing to design and implement your own Body Engineering project is extremely significant. It demonstrates the determination, creativity, and sense of responsibility essential for success.

CHAPTER SEVEN

A Troubleshooting Guide

Common Questions and Answers About Health and Fitness

To assist you in dealing with some of the concerns and problems you may encounter as you work your way through your renovation process, here are the questions most commonly asked by body engineers.

Q: *I travel a lot. How do I keep in shape on the road?*

A: Most major midlevel to high-end hotels and motor inns now offer at least basic workout facilities. A quick check with hotel personnel will tell you where it's safe to run, or if there is an accessible gym nearby. The folks at the front desk can also steer you to restaurants that serve something other than two-pound steaks or greasy fast food.

Q: *Any tips for ordering food in restaurants?*

A: Choose broiled or baked instead of fried, steamed vegetables instead of those drenched in butter or cheese, and white wine instead of Tennessee sippin' whiskey. Always ask your server if the food you are ordering can be prepared without salts (especially MSG) or oils. Season your food yourself rather than having it come to you laced with additives. Ask for oregano, parsley, onions, lemon wedges, low-sodium soy sauce, red pepper sauce (Tabasco), and mustard.

Q: *Do men exercise differently than women? Should they?*

A: Traditionally, men have wanted large biceps and bulging pecs and have used heavy resistance training to get them. Women typically have used toning routines to focus on problem areas such as the hips, lower abs, and buttocks. Exercises that isolate these areas are obviously different. Anatomically speaking, however, men and women have pretty much the same musculature. Both sexes can (and do) train with the same exercises.

Q: *I've been weight training for several months and I am becoming much stronger. My only complaint is that I'm not losing as much weight as I'd like. Am I doing something wrong?*

A: Weight training isolates the most functional cellular structure in the body—muscle tissue. The usual result of weight training is muscle development. Since muscle by volume weighs more than fat, a better gauge of your progress is your body composition. Your fat-to-muscle ratio will tell you if your workouts are burning the fat you're seeking to shed. Don't rely exclusively on the scale. If you do discover that resistance training isn't oxidizing enough fat, increase the length and intensity of your aerobic workouts.

Q: *Does weight training always make your muscles larger and heavier?*

A: Not if you don't want it to. Resistance training has almost limitless applications. After decades of research, we now know how to use weight training for total body toning, fat reduction, expansion of aerobic capability, flexibility, coordination, enhancement of muscle strength, size, and endurance, and all the other aspects of physical fitness. Not long ago, boxers weren't allowed to train with weights because their coaches believed they'd lose speed and agility. The same restrictions were thought to apply to gymnasts, figure skaters, and martial artists. Now almost all athletes in all sports rely on some sort of weight training. By changing resistance levels, degree of intensity, and number of repetitions, weight training can help everyone reach his or her fitness goals, regardless of what those goals may be.

Q: *I began weight training recently and I'm pretty sore. Am I lifting too much?*

A: Probably not. When you initially attempt to establish a resistance training routine, your body is unaccustomed to the stress involved and reacts by becoming stiff and sore. In addition, a natural defense mechanism within your muscles often retains fluids to lubricate and insulate sore muscles and stiff joints. Bear with these side effects—they're temporary. Your discomfort will subside when your body acclimates itself to your new activities. If your discomfort does not go away, try lowering the size of the weights you are lifting. Experiment and find your comfort level.

Q: *If I abandon my exercise routine, will my muscles eventually turn into fat?*

A: There's no known biochemical reaction that converts muscle to fat. What happens when you stop exercising is your metabolism slows down and, of course, you burn fewer calories each day. Those muscles you developed back in the days when you liked and respected yourself eventually begin to atrophy because they're rarely used. Weaker, smaller muscles mean fewer fat-burning mechanisms. The fat that may appear when you stop exercising isn't made of your old muscles, it replaces them.

Q: *I dramatically reduced my fat intake quite some time ago, but I haven't noticed any significant reduction in my weight. What's going on?*

A: We live in an era of no-fat and low-fat foods, and in the past five years we Americans have actually cut down on fat consumption. But during the same period, we've become more obese because most of us have replaced the fat we used to eat with high-carbohydrate foods such as cereals, rice, grains, and pasta. Carbohydrates are packed with energy. If that energy isn't burned, it will eventually be stored as body fat. So forget the low-fat magic promised by the processed-food industry. Eat a balanced diet, with adequate protein, and design an activities plan you can live with.

Q: *Which kind of exercise is better, resistance training or aerobics?*
A: Both forms offer substantial benefits, and they work best in tandem. An ideal exercise plan establishes a balance between the two. Individual goals (what are you going to use your new body for?) may dictate an emphasis on either strength or aerobic endurance, but your body needs an adequate level of each.

Q: *What is the best time of day to exercise?*
A: Any time that is free of interruption or distraction is the standard answer. Actually, it depends on your Body Engineering goals. If you have mounted a fat-reduction campaign, exercising the first thing in the morning is probably a good idea. You'll be well into a partial fast, with nothing in your stomach and low blood sugar levels. Energy from stored fat will be almost immediately accessed to fuel your sunrise workouts. If you are attempting to build strength and body mass, consume several meals before your workout, but stop eating one to two hours before exercise. If you are already in satisfactory shape, late afternoon (when your metabolism is most active) is probably when exercise is most effective and invigorating.

Q: *What kind of exercise will best increase my metabolic rate (so that I can burn more fat)?*
A: Weight training is now recognized as the most effective method for boosting metabolic activity. Not only will you burn calories

during resistance workouts, the catabolism/anabolism cycle stimulated by weight work will oxidize stored energy (fat) for up to forty-eight hours after your workout ends.

Q: *Is weight training helpful for women?*

A: Certainly. In addition to its fat-burning capabilities, resistance exercise is the only way to effectively isolate specific muscle groups. Properly applied, weight training shapes the body beautifully. Some women are leery of weight work because they don't want a bodybuilder's physique. Don't worry. Exaggerated hypertrophy is usually the result of poor technique or overly rigorous workout routines designed to increase mass and definition. Most women can achieve the benefits of weight training by using low weights and high repetition.

Q: *Although I eat dairy products and occasionally seafood, my diet is mostly vegetarian. Am I getting enough protein and other nutrients to fuel my workouts? Should I be taking some kind of supplement?*

A: Although vegetarianism is a health-promoting practice in many respects, many vegetarians experience protein deficiency. Unless one is an expert at combining foods, the protein supplied by fruits, grains, nuts, seeds, and vegetables is often inadequate. Fortunately, protein can be supplemented quite easily without violating vegetarian principles. Look for a protein supplement that offers all the essential amino acids, and select one that can be taken both with meals and on an empty stomach.

Q: *Can I really build muscle by working out on machines, or are they useful only for toning? Are free weights a better option for adding size and strength?*

A: Free weights are the preferred vehicle for resistance training. Use of free weights removes external controls and guidance, allowing the body engineer to develop structural stability, muscle control, balance, and coordination—attributes machines simply don't enhance. That doesn't mean that you should ignore resistance machines entirely. The best approach might be to perform all basic strength exercises with free weights and then utilize machines for specific movements. A bench press is best performed with a barbell or pair of dumbbells, but to isolate the chest muscles, a "pec dec" or other chest "squeezing" apparatus is ideal. Choose the combination of exercises and machinery that most closely matches your development goals.

Q: *Running and jogging have come under a lot of fire recently, with critics often advocating "power walking" as a better aerobic alternative. Lately, traditional aerobic routines have been replaced with "low-impact" exercises and yoga classes. What is your opinion of this trend?*

A: Traditional high-impact aerobic exercise requires a much greater expenditure of effort and energy than its low impact offspring. Devotees of high impact aerobics experience a much more intense, much more vigorous workout than low impact buffs. The primary cause of the flak that high-impact exercise is generating is the injury factor. Rather than specifically condemning traditional aerobics, I believe that the red flag being raised by sports medicine experts is actually evidence that too many fitness enthusiasts are trying to do too much too soon.

I recommend a judicious blend of both forms of aerobic exercise—often during the same workout. Low-impact training is an excellent way for beginners and the poorly conditioned to involve themselves in exercise without subjecting their bodies to shock or trauma. Intermediate and advanced fitness buffs should routinely mix low- and high-impact exercise. Constantly performing only high-impact activities will almost inevitably lead to breakdown or overtraining. Adding low-impact exercise to your routines allows tiny stresses and strains to heal, instead of deteriorating into major injuries. This training method, known as cycling, allows you to benefit from the valuable intensity inherent in high-impact activity, while reducing the potential for disaster.

Q: *I experience low back pain from time to time. Does using a rowing machine aggravate this problem, or can it help strengthen my back muscles?*

A: If the technique you're using is seriously flawed, rowing can indeed cause trauma to the lower vertebrae of your spinal column. Performed correctly, however, rowing is an excellent back strengthener. Properly warm up before rowing, paying special attention to the loosening of all back, leg, and arm muscles. While rowing, maintain an upright posture, with your spinal column perpendicular to the floor. Avoid any forward lean or bending at the waist or you may pull lumbar vertebrae out of their natural position and severely stress surrounding tissues. Place most of your emphasis on the arms and legs. Pull with the biceps and push with the large muscles of the legs.

   If you follow this advice and your back remains sore, consider replacing or augmenting rowing with a stationary bike, a treadmill, or a stepper. By combining several activities in one workout, you'll expend the effort necessary to burn calories and condition muscles without forcing yourself to rely on one exercise. If your back continues to be sore, consult a health professional to ensure there isn't something wrong.

Q: *I've heard conflicting recommendations concerning the amount of exercise I need to stay in shape. How many hours a week should I exercise?*

A: "More is better" doesn't always apply to physical fitness. Each individual has his or her own needs, goals, knowledge, metabolic rate, attitude, family and career commitments, access to equipment, and motivation. In general, attempting to get the most work done in the least amount of time is an effective approach to workout scheduling.

Approach your workouts with vigor and eagerness but pay close attention to form. If you exercise correctly, your metabolism will remain active twelve to twenty-four hours after your workout ends. Unless you're a triathlete or in training for the Olympics, you should be able to limit your formal exercise sessions to three or four a week. Workouts shouldn't exceed an hour and a half. Resistance training sessions need not last more than thirty or forty-five minutes. Space your workouts throughout the week so that you generate the energy you need to make your exercise sessions worthwhile and to allow your body time to recuperate between activities.

Q: *Should I drink my protein supplement before, during, or after my workout?*

A: The best time for protein consumption is sixty to ninety minutes after exercise. Because strenuous activity depletes glucose and glycogen, the body's most pressing need after a workout is replenishment of carbohydrate levels. After your carb requirement has been met, consume your protein. It's at this point that protein is needed for the reconstruction of muscle tissue.

Q: *My two growing boys are becoming interested in weight training. Can it impede their growth or development?*

A: Yes—if the weights they're lifting are too heavy. Excessive resistance will inhibit normal skeletal growth and create a number of structural imbalances. Tell your children to use light resistance for all weight training. If your kids can't complete at least twelve repetitions with a given weight, that weight is too heavy. Concentrate on technique and muscle stamina. Size and strength will come later, evolving naturally as your sons mature.

Q: *What vitamins and supplements boost energy and enhance the benefits of exercise?*

A: The kola nut herb is an excellent source of energy. This product is a natural source of caffeine and acts as a central nervous system stimulant. Ginkgo biloba increases mental acuity and circulation. Pantocrine has been garnering marvelous reviews from Olympic coaches and is the energy source and recuperative supplement preferred by most Asian athletes. Inosine has been shown to increase athletic performance by stimulating energy production in both cardiac and skeletal muscles. Try these substances one at a time, and proceed slowly. Allow yourself time to analyze the effects of each product and to decide which works best for you.

Q: *What's circuit training and what can it do for me?*
A: In conventional weight training, each set of exercises is preceded by a rest period. In circuit training, you perform an exercise, then immediately move on to another, and another, until your workout is complete. Circuit training exercises are sequenced in combinations that isolate single muscles, regional muscle groups, or the entire body. The routines preserve the toning and strength-enhancing benefits of conventional resistance training and add an aerobic element to condition your cardiorespiratory system.

Q: *Should I warm up before my exercise routine?*
A: Absolutely. Warming the body in a general fashion helps to increase heart rate and core body temperature without testing the elasticity of tissues. Use five to twenty minutes of walking, biking, jogging, or any low-stress activity to prepare your body for exercise.

Q: *I have shin splints from running. How do I treat my injury?*
A: Ice massage is the best home treatment for your shin splints. Fill two Styrofoam cups with water and freeze them. Cut away the top half of the cup to expose the ice and to leave yourself a handy surface to grip. Massage your shins in an up-and-down and circular fashion. Apply pressure for a deep tissue massage. Be sure to stretch your calves, ankles, and lower legs before

and after you run. Also be sure that your sneakers provide adequate support and cushioning.

Q: *What is your opinion of all these exercise machine infomercials I see on television at least three times a day? Are any of these machines any good?*

A: Most reputable, honest manufacturers of fitness equipment also sell their products in stores. This allows you to test their wares thoroughly before you buy. If you are interested in a home exercise device, ask a fitness professional for an objective opinion before you buy.

Q: *What is the "plateau effect"?*

A: At some point in your body renovation process (usually in the intermediate stages), your progress becomes imperceptible. Your body has adjusted to the consistent demands of your exercise routine, and needs new challenges to inspire continued improvement. Generally, the best way to combat the plateau effect is to intensify your workouts. You improved rapidly at the start of your process because you had substantial improvement to make. Quick, dramatic improvements are less likely when you've already reached the point where you're doing pretty well. What you may not realize is that you are now in a position to greatly expand your activity options. Your body is straining to test its new capabilities. Go for it.

Q: *I've reached my Body Engineering goals. What the heck do I do now?*

A: Celebrate and congratulate yourself. Give yourself credit for what you've done and what you'll continue doing. Knowing that you have designed and implemented your own Body Engineering process and—most impressively—realizing that you did the work that ensured your success should be a source of pride and strength. You have created a new life with new attitudes and new values.

If you've absorbed the principles of Body Engineering, you recognize that you must keep moving forward. The Health Maintenance template in chapter 5 will assist you in the transition from the construction phase to the operational stage of your engineering effort. If you've developed the creative and curious nature common to good engineers, you're already beginning the search for your next challenge.

Products Available From JA Fitness

Videos (VHS)

Waste-to-Waist   John Abdo has developed a highly successful waist-training routine to give you that "washboard" look. Not just another simple abdominal workout, *Waste-to-Waist* benefits your oliques, hips, buttocks, thighs and lower back. In as little as 6 minutes a day, you'll develop washboard abdominals by following any one of the three routines designed for your level of fitness.
   Retail: $24.95   JA Fitness: $19.95

One-on-One Exercise   John Abdo's *One-on-One* video is a complete fitness guide specifically designed for those individuals who don't have access to fancy equipment. Performed alone or with a partner, this program offers 40 unique movements for beginner, intermediate and advanced levels. Each exercise is designed to shape muscles, increase strength and flexibility, and burn body fat.
   Retail: $24.95   JA Fitness: $19.95

Explosive Power   John Abdo competed for twelve years as an Olympic weightlifter, winning numerous championships. And now, John wants to share his sophisticated strength-training knowledge with you. In this video you'll learn total-body "explosive" movements that develop overall muscularity, coordination, stability, cardiovascular and respiratory strength, stamina, and, of course, explosive power. As a result of applying these techniques, you'll see remarkable improvements in your vertical jumps, sprinting speeds, tendon and ligament strength, and reaction times. After performing the *Explosive Power* exercises you'll watch your body become quicker, more symmetrical and athletic as you build powerful strength and burn body fat. This video is a must for all athletes and coaches.
   Retail: $24.95   JA Fitness: $19.95

Basic Principles of Weight Training   In this one-hour video, expert trainer John Abdo offers a complete guide to basic weight-training principles. Especially helpful for every beginner and intermediate, *Basic Principles of Weight Training* is also an essential reference for even the most advanced weight trainer. In this video, you'll learn how to train every body part for maximum strength and muscular development using the correct techniques and intensities. John also discusses nutrition and aerobics while providing tips on workout srategies.
   Retail: $24.95   JA Fitness: $19.95

Nutrition

All of the nutrition products endorsed by John Abdo are natural, safe, and effective. For more information about John's line of supplements, please call or write for a free catalog.

JA FITNESS
P.O. Box 363
Algonquin, IL 60102
Phone: 1-800-331-2236
Fax: 1-847-854-2358
Web site: http://www.johnabdo.com

(These products are not offered by or through
Perigee Books or The Berkley Publishing Group.)

PUMP UP WITH PERIGEE'S BODYBUILDING BOOKS

__BIGGER MUSCLES IN 42 DAYS!
  by Ellington Darden, Ph.D.   0-399-51706-5/$16.00

__THE GOLD'S GYM BOOK OF STRENGTH TRAINING
  by Ken Sprague   0-399-51863-0/$14.00

__THE GOLD'S GYM BOOK OF WEIGHT TRAINING
  by Ken Sprague   0-399-51846-0/$14.00

__LIVING LONGER STRONGER
  by Ellington Darden, Ph.D.   0-399-51900-9/$12.00

__SPORTS STRENGTH
  by Ken Sprague   0-399-51802-9/$16.95

VISIT THE PUTNAM BERKLEY BOOKSTORE CAFÉ ON THE INTERNET:
http://www.berkley.com

Payable in U.S. funds. No cash accepted. Postage & handling: $1.75 for one book, 75¢ for each additional. Maximum postage $5.50. Prices, postage and handling charges may change without notice. Visa, Amex, MasterCard call 1-800-788-6262, ext. 1, or fax 1-201-933-2316; refer to ad # 593b

**Or, check above books
and send this order form to:**
The Berkley Publishing Group
P.O. Box 12289, Dept. B
Newark, NJ 07101-5289
Please allow 4-6 weeks for delivery.
Foreign and Canadian delivery 8-12 weeks.

Bill my: ☐ Visa   ☐ MasterCard   ☐ Amex _____(expires)

Card#_____
Daytime Phone #_____ ($10 minimum)
Signature_____

Or enclosed is my: ☐ check   ☐ money order

Ship to:
Name_____
Address_____
City_____
State/ZIP_____

Book Total $_____
Applicable Sales Tax $_____
(NY, NJ, PA, CA, GST Can.)
Postage & Handling $_____
Total Amount Due $_____

Bill to: Name_____
Address_____City_____
State/ZIP_____

HEALTH AND TRAINING GUIDES
DESIGNED SPECIFICALLY FOR WOMEN

__A WOMAN'S BOOK OF STRENGTH
by Karen Andes 0-399-51899-1/$12.00

"Karen Andes is a rare combination of expertise and sensitivity.... This should have been the first fitness book ever done."—Cher
A unique, empowering guide that shows women how to mine the powers of the heart, mind, spirit, and body.

__SIX WEEK FAT-TO-MUSCLE MAKEOVER
by Ellington Darden, Ph.d. 0-399-51562-3/$10.95

A safe and healthful diet-and-exercise plan that actually changes the body's fat-to-muscle ratio. Includes menu plans, recipes, exercise routines, and inspiring before-and-after photos.

__CORY EVERSON'S FAT-FREE AND FIT
by Cory Everson with Carole Jacobs 0-399-51858-4/$15.00

Cory Everson, internationally acclaimed fitness expert and six-time Ms. Olympia, shares her secrets to a fabulous, fat-free and fit body.

__CORY EVERSON'S WORKOUT
by Corinna Everson and Jeff Everson, Ph.D. 0-399-51684-0/$15.95

An innovative fitness program from six-time Ms. Olympia and television star Cory Everson. More than 150 black-and-white photographs.